THIS BOOK IS THE PR

AF615110

STATE ______________
PROVINCE ______________
COUNTY ______________
PARISH
SCHOOL DISTRICT ______________
OTHER ______________

in spaces
to the left as
instructed

ISSUED TO	Year Used	CONDITION	
		ISSUED	RETURNED

ARTHROSCOPY OF SMALL JOINTS

edited by

MASAKI WATANABE, M.D.
Visiting Professor,
Department of Orthopedic Surgery,
Teikyo University School of Medicine,
Tokyo

IGAKU-SHOIN Tokyo・New York

Published and distributed by
IGAKU-SHOIN Ltd.,
5-24-3 Hongo, Bunkyo-ku, Tokyo
IGAKU-SHOIN Medical Publishers, Inc.,
1140 Avenue of the Americas, New York, N.Y. 10036

Library of Congress Cataloging in Publication Data

Main entry under title:

Arthroscopy of small joints.

Bibliography: p.
Includes index.
1. Arthroscopy. 2. Joints—Diseases—Diagnosis.
I. Watanabe, Masaki. [DNLM: 1. Arthroscopy—methods.
2. Joint Diseases—diagnosis. WE 300 A7873]
RC933.A666 1985 616.7′207545 85-217
ISBN 0-89640-114-6 (New York)
ISBN 4-260-14114-7 (Tokyo)

Printed and bound in Japan

Preface

Although neglected for many years, today arthroscopy of the knee joint is being used world wide. For a time it seemed that arthroscopy of joints other than the knee could never become a clinical reality because examination of them required an extremely thin endoscope with a very close field of vision—thus the collective term "small joint arthroscopy." The development of our No. 24 (Selfoc) arthroscope in 1970 has allowed some progress toward wider clinical application of small joint arthroscopy. In this book we have presented some of our basic studies as well as clinical material—general principles indications, complications and arthroscopy of each joint.

Many problems are yet to be solved in the arthroscopy of small joints, but perhaps, with continued research, clinical trials and a serious exchange of information among arthroscopists, this application will one day reach the same level of success as knee arthroscopy.

Finally, I wish to express my great appreciation to Dr. Jo Sakakibara, who prepared the index for this book.

March 1, 1985

Masaki Watanabe, M.D.

Contributors

Yung-Cheng Chen, M.D.	Department of Orthopedic Surgery, Teikyo University School of Medicine, 2–11–1 Kaga, Itabashi-ku, Tokyo 173
Soichi Fujii, M.D.	Department of Orthopedic Surgery, Tokyo Teishin Hospital, 2–14–23 Fujimi, Chiyoda-ku, Tokyo 102
Hiroshi Ikeuchi, M.D.	Department of Orthopedic Surgery, Tokyo Teishin Hospital, 2–14–23 Fujimi, Chiyoda-ku, Tokyo 102
Kazutada Ito, M.D., D.Med.Sc.	Associate Professor, Department of Anatomy, Faculty of Medicine, Kyoto University, Yoshida Konoe-cho, Sakyo-ku, Kyoto 606; Department of Orthopedic Surgery, Kyoto University Hospital, 53 Shogoin Kawaramachi, Sakyo-ku, Kyoto 606
Ken-Ichiro Murakami, D.D.S., D.Med.Sc.	Department of Oral and Maxillofacial Surgery, Faculty of Medicine, Kyoto University, 53 Shogoin Kawaramachi, Sakyo-ku, Kyoto 606
Hitomi Nagai, M.D.	Department of Orthopedic Surgery, Tokyo Teishin Hospital, 2–14–23 Fujimi, Chiyoda-ku, Tokyo 102
Jo Sakakibara, M.D.	Associate Professor, Department of Orthopedic Surgery, Teikyo University School of Medicine, 2–11–1 Kaga, Itabashi-ku, Tokyo 173
Masaki Watanabe, M.D.	Visiting Professor, Department of Orthopedic Surgery, Teikyo University School of Medicine, 2–11–1 Kaga, Itabashi-ku, Tokyo 173
Kazuaki Yajima, M.D.	Department of Orthopedic Surgery, Tokyo Teishin Hospital, 2–14–23 Fujimi, Chiyoda-ku, Tokyo 102

Contents

I

EQUIPMENTS AND PROCEDURES

1

Equipments and Procedures of Small Joint Arthroscopy

DEFINITION OF SMALL JOINTS

From the viewpoint of arthroscopy, all joints other than the knee can be classified as "small" joints. Although the shoulder and the hip joints might be considered large joints, and the elbow and the ankle joints of medium size, arthroscopic examination of these joints requires an extremely small-gauge arthroscope. This is because the joint cavity is very narrow as compared with that of the knee joint, making introduction of the arthroscope very difficult. For this reason, the authors here refer to these joints as small joints, together with the temporomandibular acromioclavicular, wrist, metacarpophalangeal, proximal interphalangeal, and distal interphalangeal joints.

Of course, each joint has its own size and structure, and it is expected that in the future special arthroscopes will be designed for arthroscopy of each joint and for each site of the joint cavity, respectively. At present, however, one of the authors (M. W.) classifies the joints into two categories: the knee joint and the small joints. Joints other than the knee and child's joints (even the knee joint) belong to the small joints category. Also, canine knee joints in experimental arthroscopy are small joints.

HISTORY OF ARTHROSCOPY OF SMALL JOINTS

In 1931, Burman of the Hospital for Joint Diseases in New York described an arthroscopic investigation on cadaver joints. He examined about 100 knee joints, 25 shoulder joints, 15 elbow joints, 6 wrist joints, 20 hip joints, and 3 ankle joints. In most cases, the findings were checked by opening the joints. The joint cavity was distended with water, and the arthroscope he used was 3.0 mm in diameter. The total outside diameter of 4.0 mm of the sheath rendered only the knee, shoulder, and elbow joints accessible for observation. Burman stated that other joints, such as the wrist, hip, and ankle joints, should be examined by the use of a thinner arthroscope with a smaller, less oblique opening at its end. In fact, at that time, no joint other than the knee was examined on living patients through the arthroscope.

In 1939, Takagi of Tokyo University Faculty of Medicine (Fig. 1) described in his paper "The Arthroscope" his No. 1 (Fig. 2)~No. 12 arthroscopes and six cases of arthroscopy of joints other than the knee. There were four hips (two Charcot joints, one tuberculous arthritis, and one suppurative arthritis), one ankle (flail joint), and one shoulder of a patient suffering from progressive spinal muscle atrophy. Takagi also established a routine methodology for arthroscopy of the shoulder, elbow, and ankle joints. A Takagi No. 11

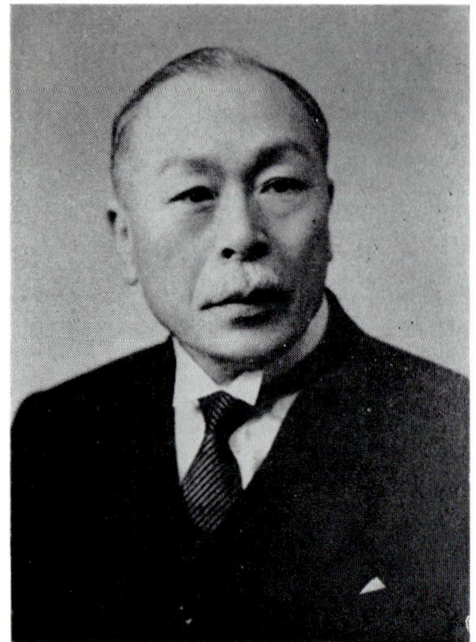

Fig. 1 Dr. Kenji Takagi.

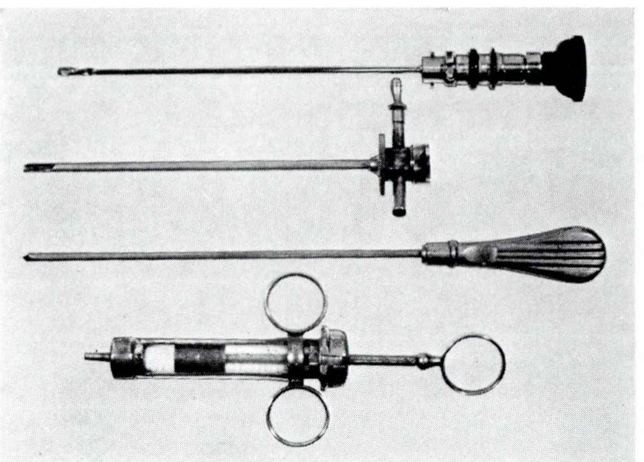

Fig. 2 Takagi No. 1 arthroscope.

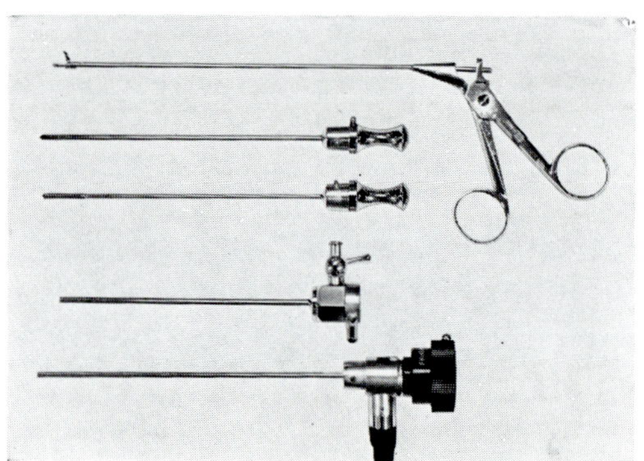

Fig. 3(a) The No. 25 arthroscope (fiberscope).

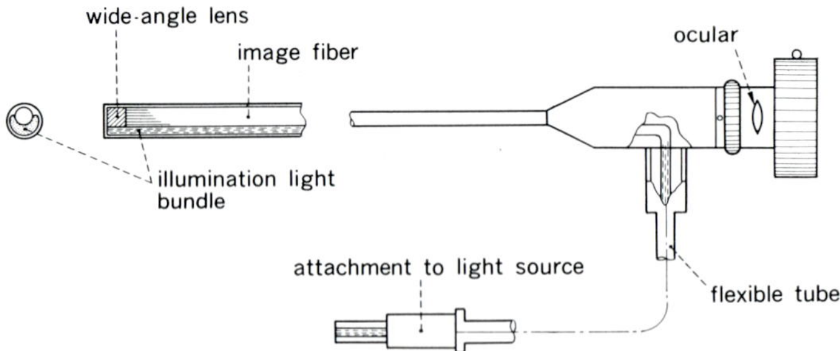

Fig. 3(b) Structure of the No. 25 arthroscope.

arthroscope with a 2.7-mm diameter was used for experimental arthroscopy of canine knee joints by Miki (1943), Koike (1943), and Okamura (1945).

For many years, one of the authors (M. W.) endeavored to develop an extremely small-gauge arthroscope to meet small joint requirements. The experiment started with the pinhole camera concept. Then a rigid, 2.0-mm diameter fiberscope (No. 23 arthroscope) and its improved type (No. 25 arthroscope) (Fig. 3a, b) were made and tested in 1967 and 1968, respectively. The fiberscopes, however, did not successfully obtain clear visualization of objects less than 3.0 mm from the tip of the scope.

All other efforts proved unsuccessful until 1968 when a new light-transmitting material named Selfoc was developed jointly by the Nippon Sheet Glass Company, Osaka, and Nippon Electric Company, Tokyo.

Selfoc, a brand name meaning "self-focusing," was first developed as laser beam-transmitting material. The author (M. W.) attempted to develop an arthroscope for small joints with a Selfoc glass rod in 1970.

ARTHROSCOPES FOR SMALL JOINT ARTHROSCOPY

Arthroscopy of small joints required the solution of many problems. First, the arthroscope must be very thin to facilitate introduction of the scope into the narrow joint space.

The arthroscope is used through a sheath, and the outside diameter of the sheath must be very thin for successful insertion into the small joint. In arthroscopy of the metacarpophalangeal joint, for instance, outside diameter of the sheath should be less than 2.0 mm. Second, it is essential that the arthroscope can be used for diagnostic purposes.

PRINCIPLE OF THE SELFOC ARTHROSCOPE

Selfoc is prepared by an ion-exchange treatment of a 1.0-mm diameter glass rod of special composition. In the Selfoc glass rod, the refractive index is greatest at the central axis and reduces gradually from its central axis to the periphery according to the following parabolic equation:

$$n = n_0\left(1 - \frac{1}{2}ar^2\right)$$

where n_0 is the refractive index at central axis, n is the refractive index at a distance r from the central axis, and a is a positive coefficient regarding the distribution of refractive index in the Selfoc.

The light beam directed to the periphery is constantly refracted back toward the central axis in the Selfoc.

On the other hand, when the light beam passes along an axis in a medium having a refractive index of n, we have the following paraxial equation:

$$\frac{d^2y}{dx^2} = \frac{1}{n} \cdot \frac{dn}{dy}$$

The equation $n = n_0\left(1 - \frac{1}{2}ar^2\right)$ can be rewritten as follows:

$$n = n_0\left(1 - \frac{1}{2}ay^2\right)$$

Consequently, the following two equations hold:

$$n = n_0\left(1 - \frac{1}{2}ay^2\right) \tag{1}$$

$$\frac{d^2y}{dx^2} = \frac{1}{n} \cdot \frac{dn}{dy} \tag{2}$$

Equation (1) differentiated in respect to y:

$$\frac{dn}{dy} = -n_0 ay \tag{3}$$

Equation (3) substituted to equation to (2):

$$\frac{d^2y}{dx^2} = -\frac{n_0}{n}ay$$

$$\frac{d^2y}{dx^2} = -ay\left(\text{provided } \frac{1}{2}ay^2 \ll 1\right) \tag{4}$$

Equation (4) is the differential equation obtained, and the solution is as follows:

$$y = A \sin \sqrt{a}\, x + B \cos \sqrt{a}\, x \tag{5}$$

Equation (5) can be transfered as follows:

$$y = C \sin (\sqrt{a}\, x + b)$$

Consequently, in the Selfoc glass rod, the light beam passes, drawing a sine curve configuration (Fig. 4a) with minimum transmission loss (0.1–0.2 dB/meter) which is less than that

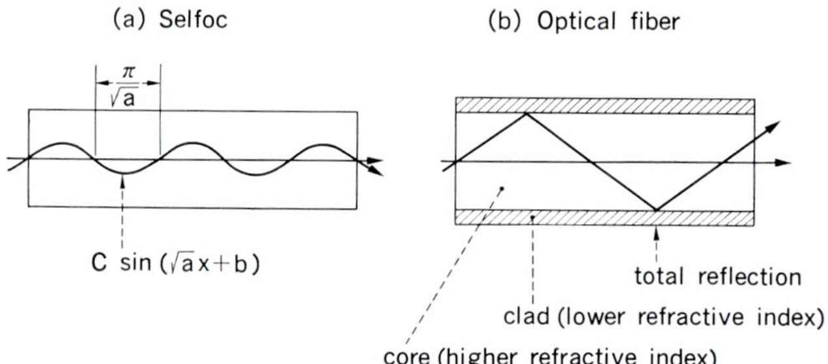

Fig. 4 Light transmission in Selfoc and optical fiber.

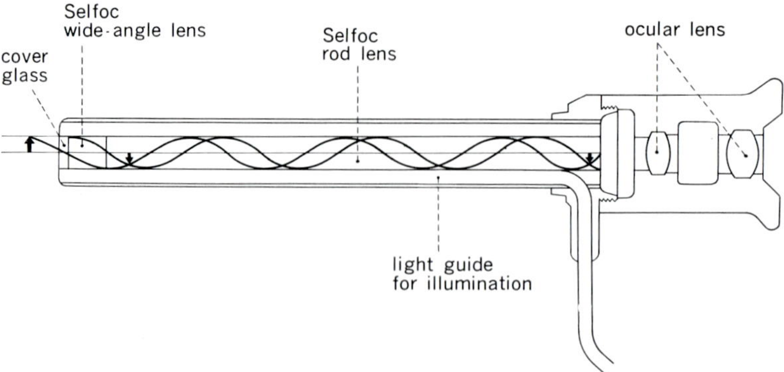

Fig. 5 Structure of No. 24 arthroscope (in early stage of development).

found in the case of optical fiber (0.7 dB/meter). In the optical fiber, the light beam proceeds repeating total reflection at the peripheral inner surface (Fig. 4b).

Furthermore, a Selfoc glass rod of suitable length has the function of a lens with a very short focal distance and a greater focal depth ranging from 1 mm to infinity, and can transmit an image as shown in Figure 5. These properties of the Selfoc arthroscope permit clear visualization of objects very close to its tip, as well as objects at a certain distance. The image standing in the surface of the cross section of the Selfoc glass rod can be magnified by the ocular attached to the Selfoc glass rod. Correction of the chromatic aberration is also achieved by means of the appropriate ocular.

Thus an object can be observed and photographed through the apparatus. This is the principle of the Selfoc arthroscope.

THE WATANABE NO. 24 ARTHROSCOPE (SELFOSCOPE)

The Selfoc arthroscope was developed for arthroscopy of small joints in 1970. The gauge of the scope was 1.7 mm in diameter and the outside diameter of the sheath was 2.0 mm. The Watanabe No. 24 arthroscope permitted observation of many small joints previously not accessible. Also, a biopsy punch and forceps were designed to be inserted and manipulated through the sheath of same size as that used for telescope.

The authors' first report of the Selfoc arthroscope was made in February 1971 at the regular meeting of Tokyo Orthopaedic Surgeons. A subsequent report on the use of the Selfoc arthroscope on 19 small joints in living patients followed in April 1971, at the 45th Annual Meeting of the Japanese Orthopaedic Association.

However, this type of Selfoc arthroscope was only the first step in the development of an endoscope for small joints. Consequently, testing continued and the instrument was improved.

The No. 24 consisted of a direct viewing telescope and a fore-oblique viewing telescope, plus accessories (Figs. 6 and 7). The visual angles were 55° and 70°, respectively. As shown in Figure 8, there was no marked difference in visual angle between the two telescopes when used in water. But fore-oblique viewing telescope may be more useful in the medium of normal saline.

From the development of the first Selfoc arthroscope in January 1970 to October 5, 1972, the device was tested on 188 joints (Table 1). It was found that brightness of the illumination and correction of the chromatic aberration were insufficient.

In 1974, the ocular of the No. 24 was improved through the combined efforts of the

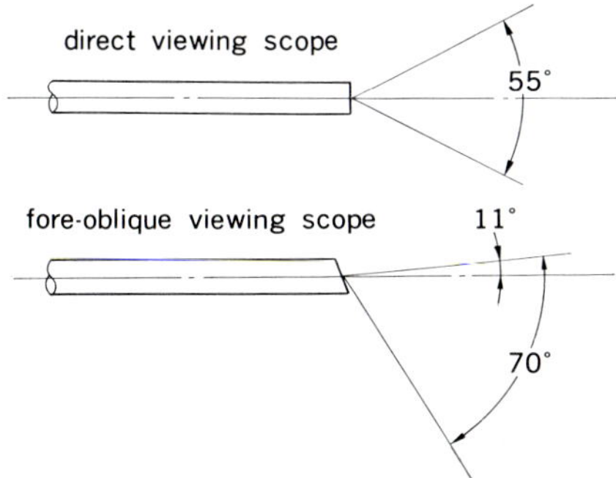

Fig. 6 Direct viewing and fore-oblique viewing telescopes.

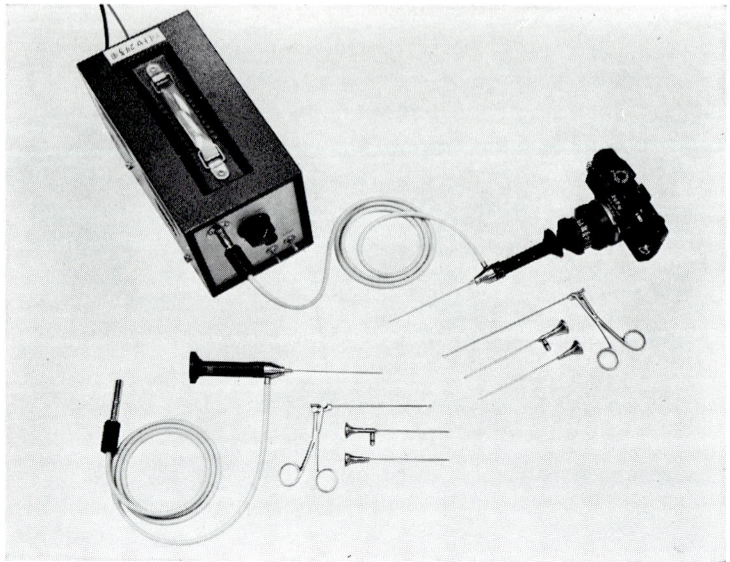

Fig. 7 No. 24 arthroscope kit.

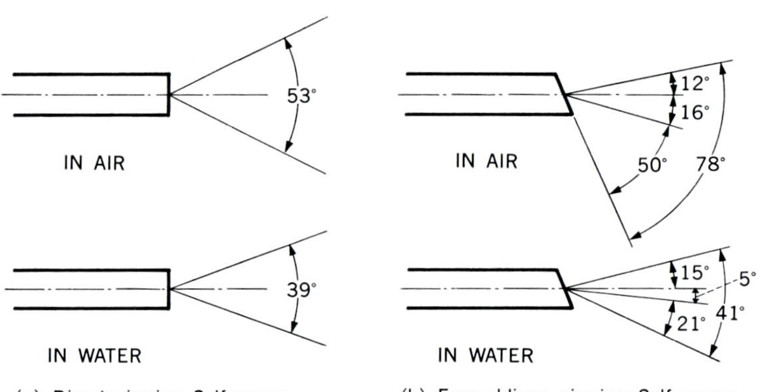

Fig. 8 Field of vision of No. 24 arthroscope.

Olympus Optical Company, Tokyo, and the Department of Orthopedic Surgery of Tokyo Teishin Hospital, Tokyo. Consequently, the illumination and correction of chromatic aberration reached a satisfactory level. This improved type of the No. 24 arthroscope was named "Selfoscope" by the Olympus Optical Company. The structure of the Selfoscope is shown in Figure 9. The 1.0-mm diameter Selfoc glass rod lens is coated with 0.25-mm thick layer of optical fibers. Set in a stainless steel tube, the total outside diameter of the device is 1.7 mm.

A No. 24 Arthroscope (Selfoscope) Kit

A complete Watanabe No. 24 arthroscope (Selfoscope) kit (Fig. 10) includes a direct viewing scope with a 125-cm long glass fiber light guide and a fore-oblique viewing scope of the same size as the direct viewing telescope; one light unit with cord; two sheaths with outside diameters of 2.0 mm and 2.3 mm, respectively, plus a needle and an obturator; and a biopsy punch and forceps. Also included are a camera body and an appropriate attach-

Table 1 Joints examined with the No. 24 arthroscope (January 1970 to October 5, 1972)

Joints examined	Number
Acromioclavicular joint	2
Shoulder joint (including subacromial bursa)	10
Elbow joint	38
Wrist joint	21
Distal radioulnar joint	3
First carpometacarpal joint	1
Metacarpophalangeal joint	21
Interphalangeal and proximal interphalangeal joints	4
Hip joint (adult)	8
Hip joint (child's)	16
Ankle joint	28
Metatarsophalangeal joint	5
Tendon sheath, bursa	3
(Subtotal—joints other than knee	160)
Knee joint	28
Total	188

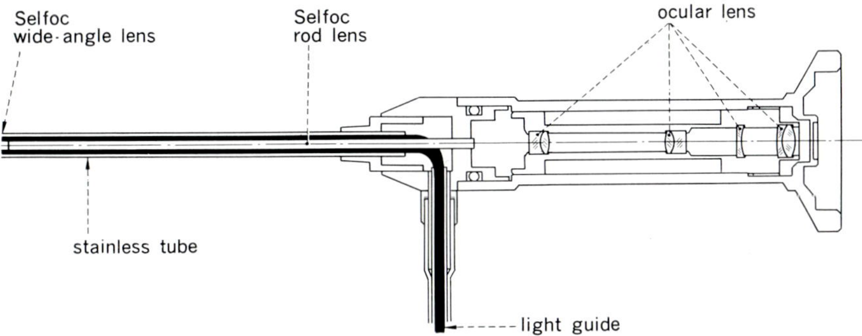

Fig. 9 Structure of the new No. 24 (Selfoscope) with improved ocular.

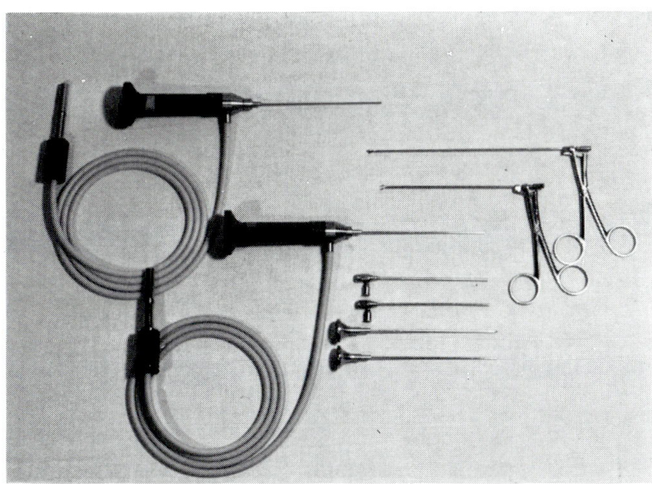

Fig. 10 No. 24 arthroscope.

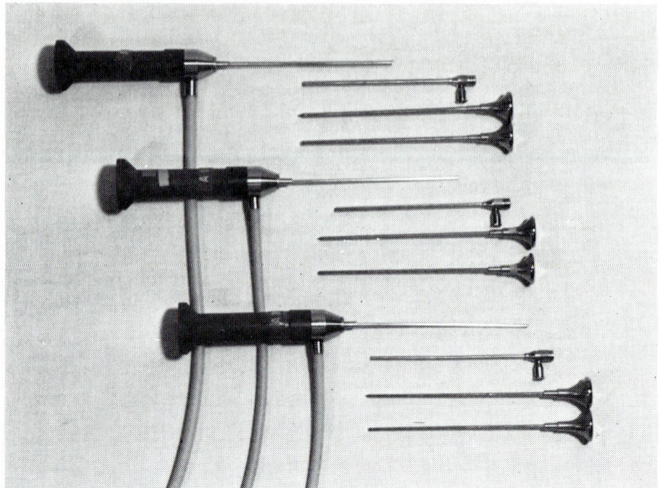

Fig. 11 No. 24-B, 24-C, and 24-D arthroscopes.

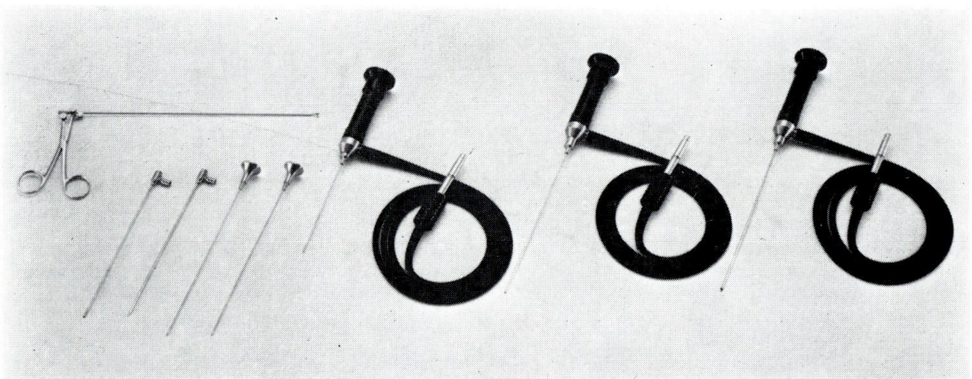

Fig. 12 Three types of Selfoscopes, 1.7 mm in diameter, and accessory instruments.

ment for the scope, plus a 30.0 cm silicon tube for supplying normal saline during arthroscopy.

The No. 24-B, No. 24-C, and No. 24-D scopes (Fig. 11) were recently added to the No. 24 arthroscope kit.

As shown in Table 2, the original Selfoscope was 1.7 mm in diameter. Next, three Selfoscopes in different sizes—2.2 mm, 2.7 mm, and 3.2 mm in diameter were tested for small joint arthroscopy. The 2.2-mm diameter Selfoscope was found suitable for arthroscopy of small joints other than finger joints. The 2.2-mm diameter scope is used through the 2.5-mm outside diameter sheath, and is not as fragile as the original Selfoscope.

Consequently, both 1.7-mm and 2.2-mm diameter Selfoscopes were found practical, and Olympus Optical Company produced two units of Selfoscope, each of which has direct viewing, fore-oblique viewing, and side viewing scopes, respectively (Fig. 12), (Table 3).

Each Selfoscope has a Selfoc glass rod of 1.0 mm in diameter. The difference in the diameter of the Selfoscope is due to the amount of optical fibers set in the Selfoscope.

Arthroscopy of the small joints has become possible through the use of Selfoscopes de-

Table 2 Different sizes of No. 24 arthroscope

	Diameter of scope	Outside diameter of sheath
24-A (Prototype)	1.7 mm	2.0 mm
24-B type	2.2 mm	2.5 mm
24-C type	2.7 mm	3.0 mm
24-D type	3.2 mm	3.5 mm

Table 3 Two different types of Selfoscopes

	Unit 1	Unit 2
Diameter of Selfoc glass rod lens	1.0 mm	1.0 mm
Diameter of optical insertion tube	1.7 mm	2.2 mm
Visual angle (in air)		
Direct viewing	55°	55°
Fore-oblique viewing	75°	75°
Side viewing	55°	55°

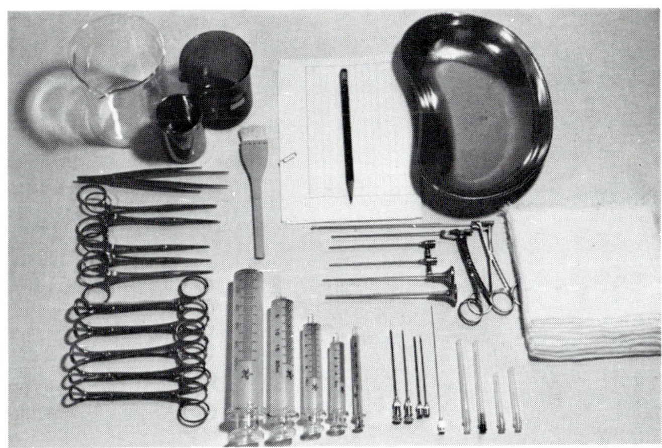

Fig. 13 Standard tray for arthroscopy.

scribed. However, it should be noted that this field differs from knee arthroscopy in some points.

Standard Tray for Arthroscopy

Trays should be designed to meet the requirements of most arthroscopy procedures to be done. One tray that meets most demands can be assembled. Such a tray (Fig. 13) includes four syringes—two 50.0 ml, one 10.0 ml, two 5.0 ml, and one tuberculin syringe. Three needles are needed on the tray—one 10.0 cm, 19 gauge; one 3.8 cm, 21 gauge; and one 3.0 cm, 23 gauge. Two glass measuring cups—a 500-ml cup for normal saline and a 100-ml cup for local anesthetic drugs—forceps, and gauze dressings complete the tray.

FUNDAMENTALS OF TECHNIQUE

Clinical arthroscopic visualization of the interior of small joints demands an accurate knowledge of the gross anatomy and pathology of each joint. There are many problems to be solved in arthroscopy of small joints, as had been the case in knee arthroscopy.

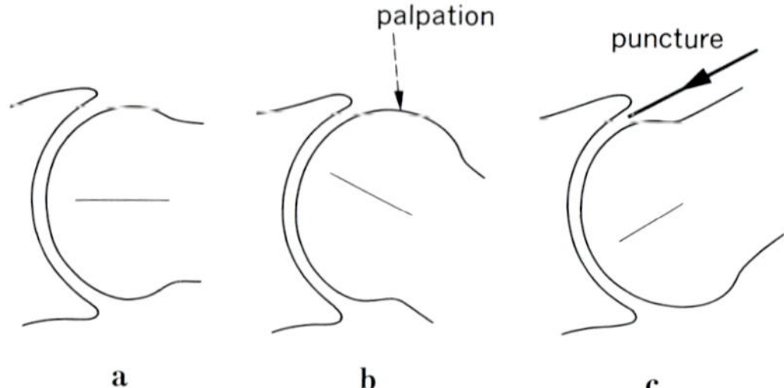

Fig. 14 Principle for joint puncture. (a) Neutral position. (b) Position for palpation of the joint space. (c) Position for insertion of an aspiration needle.

First, arthroscopy of small joints differs from knee arthroscopy in that it is impossible to observe most parts of the whole joint cavity through one puncture. In arthroscopy of the knee joint with the No. 21 arthroscope, most parts of the interior of the joint can be visualized by a lateral infrapatellar approach, while in arthroscopy of small joints, the most appropriate approach should be selected for each purpose.

The technique of arthroscopy of a small joint should be based on a knowledge of the anatomy of the joint. First of all, the technique of puncture for each joint should be learned. Here, the authors refer to the general principle of joint puncture. As shown in Figure 14, the joint space line is first palpated in a position where the convex head of the joint body is easily palpated. For instance, in the case of puncture of the wrist joint, the wrist is first held in a palmar flexed position. Repeating dorsiflexion and palmar flexion of the wrist joint while palpating the back of the wrist with the examiner's thumb facilitates easy recognition of the joint space line. After recognition of the joint space line, change to a slightly dorsiflexed position so that the convex head goes deeper into the joint space. In this position an aspiration needle is inserted toward the joint space tangentially to the convex head. The joint cavity is then filled with normal saline and distended to make trocar puncture safer.

Because of the narrowness of the joint cavity, arthroscopy of small joints should be carried out under higher fluid pressure than used in knee arthroscopy. To obtain sufficient hydrostatic pressure, it is necessary to have an assistant control the irrigating syringe instead of using a suspended bottle of normal saline or an irrigator. The authors tested the use of an automatic syringe for obtaining sufficient hydrostatic pressure in small joints, instead of the use of a suspended bottle of normal saline. Figures 15 and 16 show the relationship of the intraarticular pressure of the human elbow joint, the volume of normal saline to be injected into the joint cavity, and the intraarticular pressure in which the No. 24 arthroscope is used. As shown in the figures, the intraarticular pressure of the elbow joint during arthroscopy ranges from 70 mmHg to 200 mmHg. The best view is generally obtained at about 100 mmHg.

As the Selfoc scope is very fragile, an obturator should be used when moving the scope to other parts in the joint.

To widen the narrow joint space for better observation, manipulations such as traction, rotation, adduction, abduction, flexion, extension, pronation, and supination of the joint together with considerable distension with normal saline are necessary.

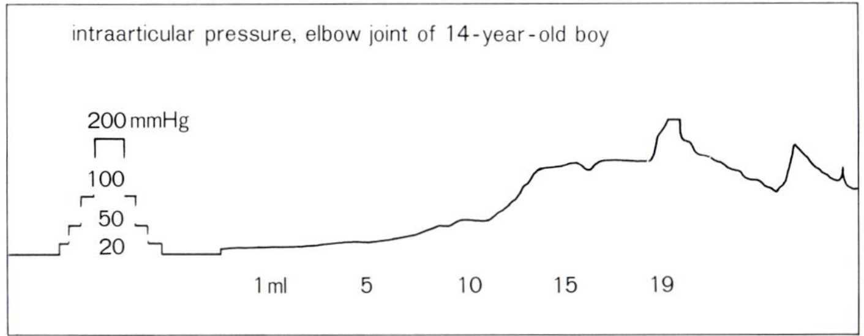

Fig. 15 Correlation of the volume of saline injected with the intraarticular pressure.

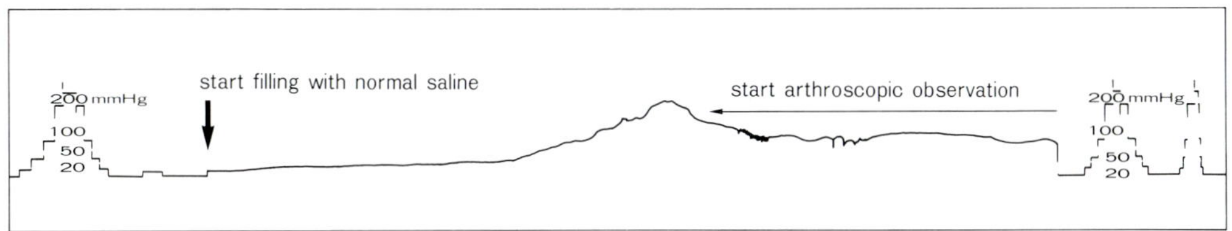

Fig. 16 Changes in intraarticular pressure during arthroscopy.

INDICATIONS

Indications for arthroscopy of joints other than the knee are:

1. Diagnosis of osteochondral fracture, osteochondritis dissecans, loose bodies, or some kinds of arthritis as well as judging the degree and extent of pathological changes in rheumatoid joints
2. Diagnosis of the intraarticular fracture of child's elbow joint and confirming of the reposition
3. Observation of lunate bone in Kienböck's disease and femoral head in congenital dislocation of the hip joint
4. Diagnosis of lesions in the shoulder joint such as lesion in glenoidal labrum, rupture of biceps longus tendon, lesion in the cuff, and Banker's lesion
5. Observation of the intraarticular condition of the hip joint of congenital dislocation
6. For arthroscopic surgery

The No. 24 is used also in knee arthroscopy for observation of some areas difficult to see with other arthroscopes such as the popliteal cavity, posterior edge of the medial meniscus, undersurface of the menisci, and child's knee joint.

COMPLICATIONS

There are several problems to be discussed with regard to complications pursuant to arthroscopy of small joints, as is the case with knee arthroscopy.

Infection

As an infection might occur as a complication of arthroscopy, strict aseptic care similar to that in any surgical operation on the joint is essential. To date, however, after more than 1,000 experiences, we have not had a single instance of suppuration after arthroscopy of small joints.

Injuries to the Cartilage and Capsules of the Joint

Injuries to the cartilaginous surface can be prevented if the joint cavity is amply distended with normal saline and trocar puncture is made gently. When moving the sheath from one point to another in the joint, an obturator should be used instead of a trocar.

Trocar puncture produces a hole in the capsule that heals, leaving a small scar in the capsule. Pain in the region of the scar is rare and temporary.

Injuries to Nerves, Tendons, and Blood Vessels

Care must be taken to avoid injuries to nerves, tendons, and blood vessels by puncture procedure. Injury to the cephalic vein in shoulder puncture, ulnar nerve in ulnar elbow puncture, extensor pollicis longus tendon in rheumatoid wrist joint puncture, dorsal artery of foot in ankle joint puncture, and so on must be especially guarded against.

Local Edema

As the joint cavity is very narrow, it is necessary to strongly distend the joint cavity with normal saline. Therefore, periarticular edema is unavoidable. The edema disappears within a few hours.

Intraarticular Bleeding and Hemarthrosis

Bleeding by trocar puncture usually stops very soon and does not disturb the clear image during arthroscopy if the joint cavity is washed several times with normal saline. Hemarthrosis after arthroscopy is seldom extensive enough to necessitate treatment. As bleeding with punch biopsy is inevitable, the joint cavity is washed several times with normal saline before withdrawal of the sheath and hemostatic agents may be injected if necessary.

In some cases of punch biopsy, a small amount of brown bloody effusion may be aspirated one week after the biopsy. This usually disappears within a few weeks through gentle washing of the joint with normal saline once a week. Traumatic arthritis resulting from arthroscopic procedure is rare and of short duration.

Accidents during Arthroscopy

Accidents during arthroscopy are similar to those during knee arthroscopy. As a 1.7-mm diameter Selfoc arthroscope is very fragile, care must be taken to manipulate it very gently in the joint.

PREOPERATIVE CONSIDERATIONS

General Information

All patients should have a complete, routine history taken and should undergo physical examination with laboratory tests prior to arthroscopy.

Oral Intake

When anesthesia other than local anesthesia is to be used, intake of fluids and solids by mouth should be restricted for at least six hours before arthroscopy.

Asepsis

Sterilization of the instrument and aseptic technique are similar to that used in knee arthroscopy. The examination should be carried out in an operating room under strict aseptic procedures similar to those used for any surgery of the joint. The telescopes with light guide, camera body, attachment for the telescope, and silicon tube should be sterilized by 24 hours exposure to formalin vapor.

The patient's skin should be prepared with one of the routine surgical preparations. The authors use 5% iodine solution and aqueous thimerosal (Merthiolate).

ANESTHESIA

Arthroscopy of small joints is usually performed under local anesthesia and/or intra-articular anesthesia. However, general or conducting anesthesia is also used. General anesthesia is common for arthroscopy of children's joints; spinal or epidural anesthesia for hip arthroscopy and Kulenkampff's anesthesia for shoulder joint arthroscopy are also used in some cases.

Local Infiltration Anesthesia

A weal is raised with a 23-gauge needle, and a larger needle is used to inject the main bulk of solution through this weal. For painless skin puncture, infiltration should be intra-dermal as well as subcutaneous. A slow, gentle technique is important, and the solution should be sufficiently injected into the fibrous layer of the joint capsule.

General, spinal, and epidural anesthesia, peripheral nerve block, or intracapsular block may be used in certain cases. General anesthesia is preferred for children.

Local anesthetic drugs now generally used include procaine (Novocain), lidocaine (Xylocaine), tetracaine (Pontocaine), mepivacaine (Carbocaine), and bupivacaine (Marcaine). Although an average and maximum dosage for each drug can be given, dosage should be varied according to the patient's age, physical condition, and complicating diseases. The main concern in local anesthesia is not exceeding the toxic dose of the local anesthetic agent (Table 4).

Puncture and Filling the Joint Cavity with Normal Saline

The joint cavity is filled and distended with normal saline or a local anesthetic drug to make the trocar puncture safer. As with insertion of an aspiration needle, the trocar sheath is inserted into the joint space. Normal saline flowing out of the sheath when the trocar is pulled out indicates that the point of the sheath lies in the joint space.

The trocar puncture is most important step in arthroscopy of small joints. Puncture of a small joint should be done carefully and gently to prevent injuries to cartilage (Fig. 17).

Arthroscopy of small joints can be performed without skin incision and without the

Table 4 Maximum dosage of each anesthetic agent

Drug	Trademark	Maximum Dosage
Procaine	Novocaine	200 ml of 0.5% = 1,000 mg 100 ml of 1.0% = 1,000 mg
Tetracaine	Pontocaine	1 mg per pound body weight not to exceed 200 mg
Lidocaine	Xylocaine	100 ml of 0.5% = 500 mg 50 ml of 1.0% = 500 mg
Mepivacaine	Carbocaine	100 ml of 0.5% = 500 mg 50 ml of 1.0% = 500 mg
Bupivacaine	Marcaine	1 mg per pound body weight not to exceed 200 mg

From Moore, D. C.: Regional Block, 4th ed., Charles C Thomas Publisher, Springfield, Illinois, 1969. Used by permission from the author and publisher.

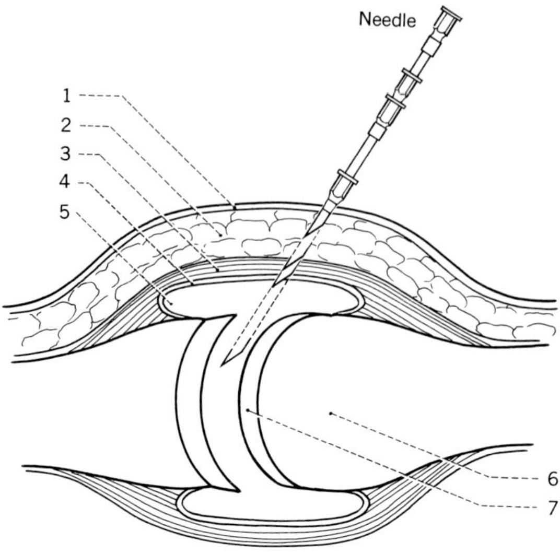

Fig. 17 Aspiration of articular fluid. (1) Skin. (2) Subcutaneous tissue. (3) Capsular ligament. (4) Synovialis. (5) Joint cavity. (6) Head. (7) Articular cartilage.

use of a tourniquet. However, a small, 2-mm long skin incision is good for gentle trocar puncture, and a tourniquet can be used when necessary.

The irrigation system is then attached to the connector of the sheath. The joint cavity is filled with normal saline discharged from a syringe controlled by an assistant, while the operator simultaneously closes the sheath with his or her thumb. The patient usually feels the joint swelling because of the increasing pressure. The cock of the irrigation tube is closed, the trocar is pulled out, and the telescope is nested within the sheath. The light guide is attached to the light unit and the transformer is switched on. Thus the stage is set for observation. The examination is carried out under continuous irrigation with normal saline by an assistant.

ARTHROSCOPY OF EACH JOINT

Arthroscopy of each joint should be based on arthroscopic anatomy of that joint. Arthroscopic anatomy should first be investigated on the joint of a dissected or amputated limb; second on the joint of a cadaver. The arthroscopic findings are checked by opening the joint. Arthroscopy is then applied to the joints on clinical cases.

In arthroscopy of the shoulder joint of a dissected limb, for instance, the joint cavity can be expanded with 100 ml of water, so that detailed observation is much easier than in undissected joints. Figures 18 through 21 and 26 are arthroscopic views of a shoulder joint of dissected limb photographed by Dr. R. Vatanachai.

From the development of the first Selfoc arthroscope in 1970 to March 31, 1980, the authors used the device in Tokyo Teishin Hospital on a total of 1,202 joints (847 joints other than the knee and 355 knee joints) (Table 5). A tendon sheath and three bursas were also examined by the use of the Selfoc arthroscope. In the following section, the authors briefly explain their experience in arthroscopy of each joint by use of Selfoc arthroscopes in the first stage of their development.

Details of arthroscopy of each joint will be discussed in Chapters 4 through 10.

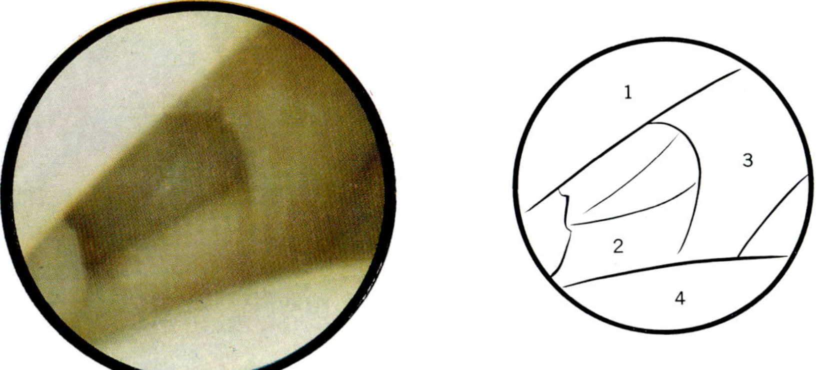

Fig. 18 Left shoulder joint, posterior approach. (1) Biceps. (2) Middle glenohumeral ligament. (3) Subscapularis. (4) Humeral head. (Courtesy of Dr. R. Vatanachai.)

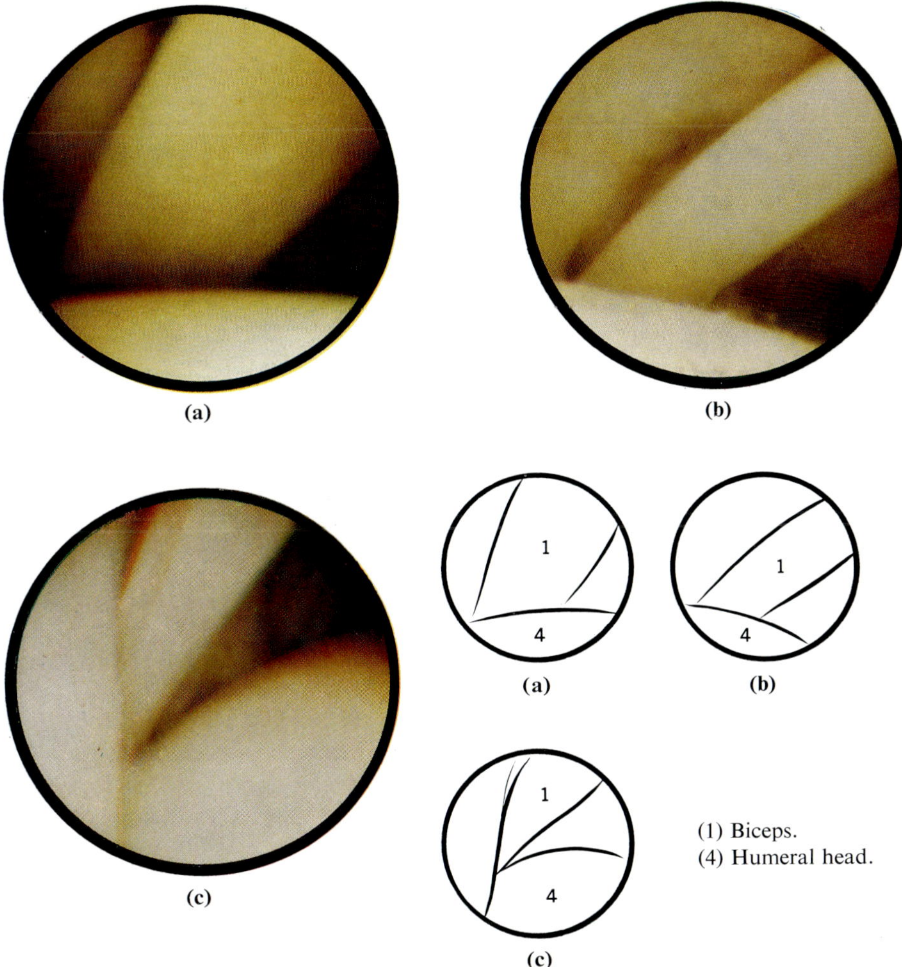

(1) Biceps.
(4) Humeral head.

Fig. 19 Normal biceps tendon of the left shoulder joint, posterior approach. (Courtesy of Dr. R. Vatanachai.)

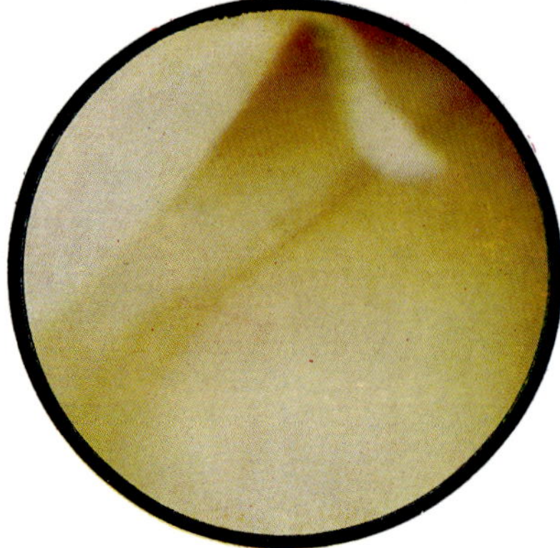

Fig. 20 Anterior glenoid labrum of the left shoulder joint. (Courtesy of Dr. R. Vatanachai.)

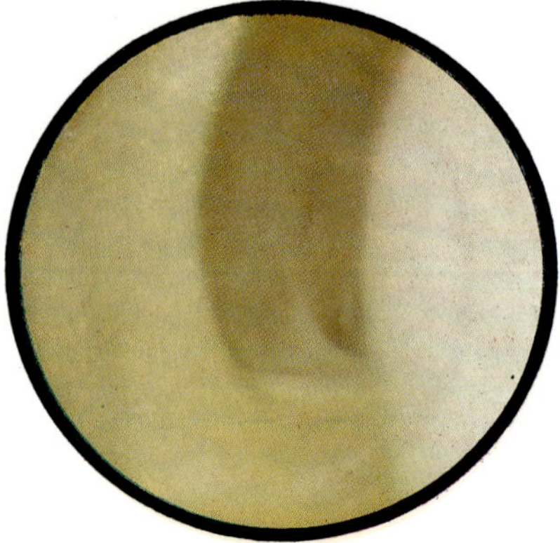

Fig. 21 Interior pouch of the left shoulder joint, anterior approach. (Courtesy of Dr. R. Vatanachai.)

Table 5 Joints examined with the No. 24 arthroscope (January 1970 to March 31, 1980)

Joint examined	Number
Temporomandibular joint	2
Acromioclavicular joint	5
Shoulder joint	123
Elbow joint	179
Wrist joint	100
First carpometacarpal joint	3
Metacarpophalangeal joint	66
Interphalangeal and proximal interphalangeal joints	16
Distal interphalangeal joint	1
Hip joint	99
Ankle joint	236
Metatarsophalangeal joint	17
(Subtotal—joints other than knee	847)
Knee joint	355
Total	1,202

Shoulder Joint

Insertion of the No. 24-A or No. 24-B scope into the joint is possible. Usually anterior and posterior approaches are required for visualization of the shoulder joint.

For arthroscopy of the right shoulder, the patient is placed on the left side. Anteriorly, the puncture is made just lateral to the coracoid process with the instrument directed toward the anterior joint line (Fig. 22a). Care must be taken to avoid injury to the cephalic vein. The anterior joint space is relatively wide, and observation here is made with rotation, abduction, or traction of the arm. By means of the Selfoc arthroscope, the anterosuperior two thirds of the humeral head, a part of the glenoid fossa, as well as the humeral course of the long head of the biceps tendon can be seen. The origin of the tendon is covered by fatty villi.

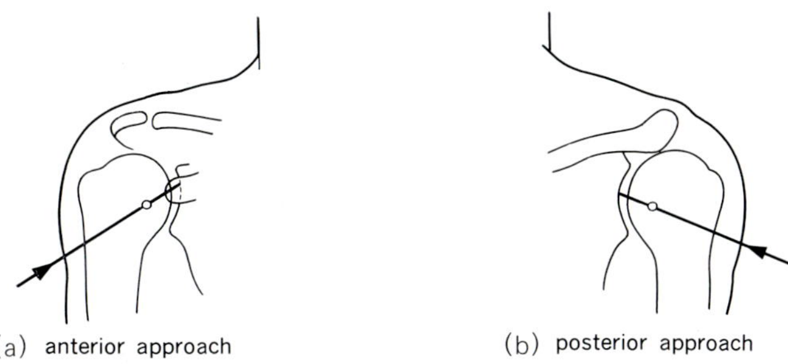

Fig. 22 Anterior and posterior approaches for visualization of the shoulder joint.

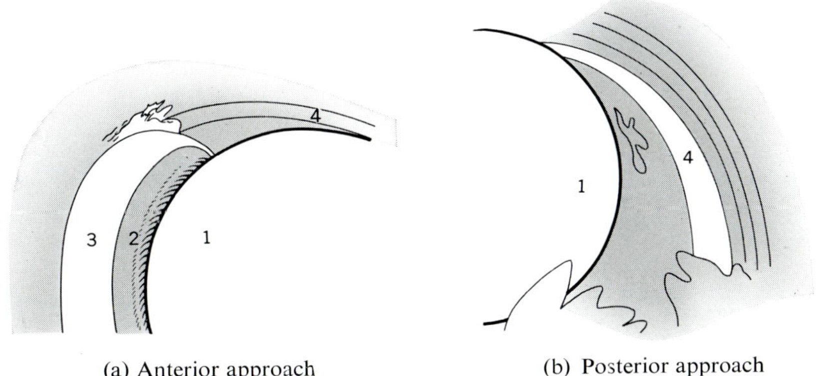

Fig. 23 Arthroscopic views of the shoulder joint, left shoulder. See also Fig. 24. (1) Head of the humerus. (2) Glenoidal fossa. (3) Labrum. (4) Tendon of the biceps long head.

Posteriorly, the trocar is inserted at a point 3 cm below the lateral inferior angle of the acromion, and the tip of the instrument is directed toward the apex of the coracoid process (Fig. 22b). The posterior and superior two thirds of the humeral head, as well as the glenoid fossa and labrum can be seen. Also the long head of the biceps tendon can be seen, although it is partially obscured by fat as it courses along the cartilaginous surface of the humeral head (Fig. 23). Examples are shown in Figures 24 through 27.

In both the anterior and posterior approaches, villi may interfere with the observation of the cartilaginous surface, and the inferior aspect of the joint is difficult to see by the usual approach methods. In such a case, a more inferior approach should be chosen.

Acromioclavicular Joint

Arthroscopy of the acromioclavicular joint is possible only when it is dislocated or becomes swollen (Fig. 28).

Elbow Joint

Because of complexity of its structure, arthroscopy of the elbow joint requires use of two or more of the six available routes (Fig. 29).

The patient lies in the dorsal recumbent position, or a lateral position is employed. The operator stands at the side of the patient, who is usually placed on his or her right or left

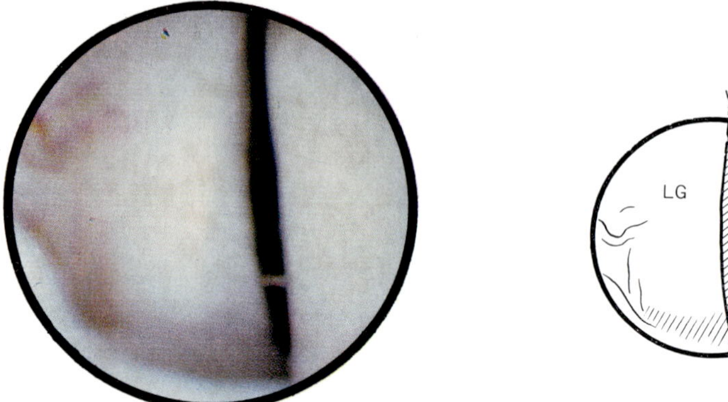

Fig. 24 A 24-year-old man with pain in the shoulder joint, posterior approach. (H) humeral head. (LG) labrum glenoidale.

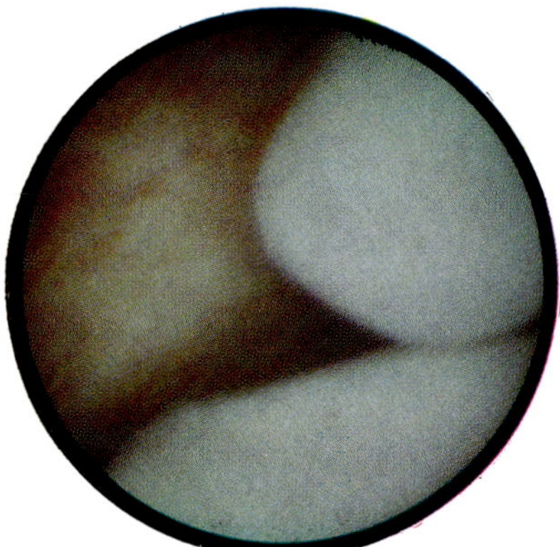

Fig. 25 A 65-year-old woman with rheumatoid arthritis. Loose bodies are observed in the left shoulder joint.

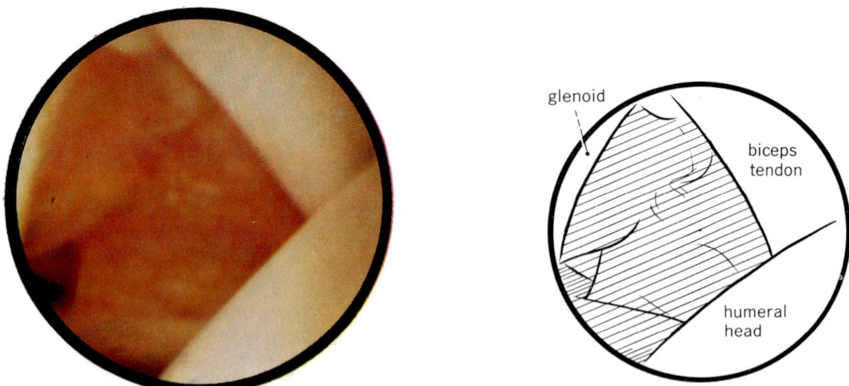

Fig. 26 A 15-year-old boy with right shoulder pain when throwing. Arthroscopically, no pathological finding is seen. (Courtesy of Dr. R. Vatanachai.)

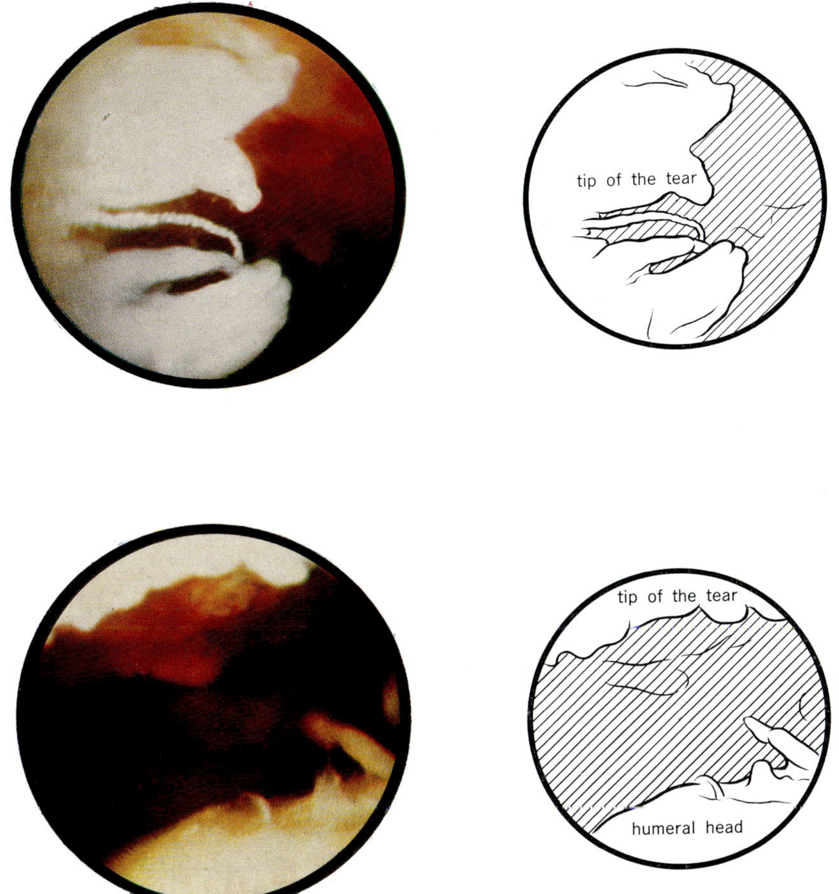

Fig. 27 A 61-year-old man with tear of the rotator cuff of the right shoulder.(Courtesy of Dr. H. Tsutsui, Tokyo.)

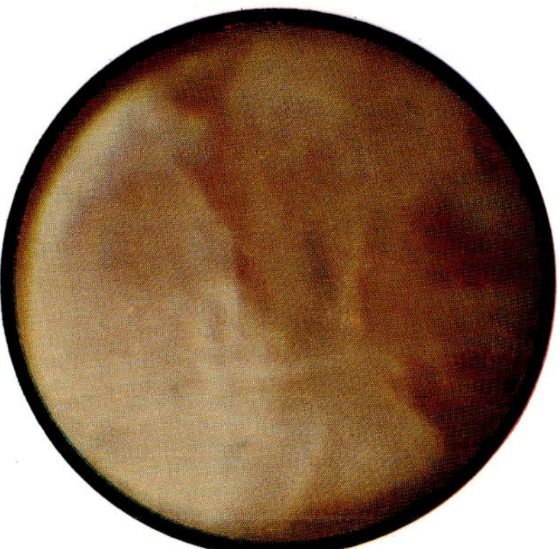

Fig. 28 A 59-year-old man with inflammatory villi of the right acromioclavicular joint.

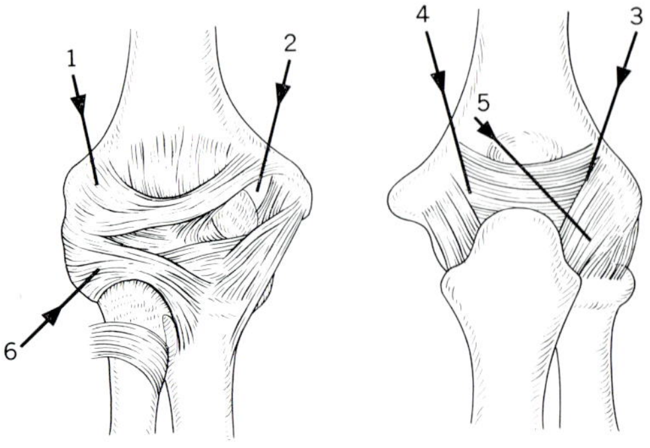

Fig. 29 Approaches to the elbow joint. (1) Supracondylar anterior radial approach. (2) Supracondylar anterior ulnar approach. (3) Supraolecranal radial approach. (4) Supraolecranal ulnar approach. (5) Posterior radial approach. (6) Anterior radial approach.

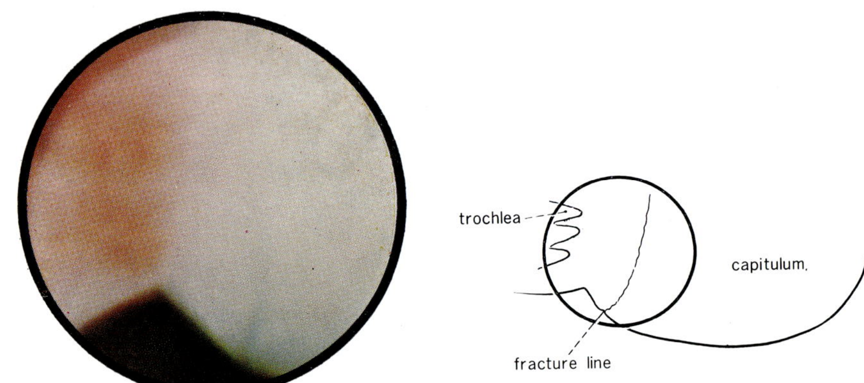

Fig. 30 A 4-year-old girl with fracture of the lateral condyle of the left humerus. Reduction of fracture dislocation was confirmed arthroscopically by supracondylar anterior radial approach.

side with the knees flexed, the upper arm at the side, and the forearm flexed at an appropriate angle to the arm. The point of puncture is chosen for each approach.

In an arthritic elbow joint, villi—especially edematous villi—may interfere with the observation of the joint surface. In performing an anterior approach, the trocar should be pointed dorsally to avoid injury to the major blood vessels. In the supraolecranal ulnar approach, care must be exercised to avoid injury of the ulnar nerve. Manipulation of the arm in flexion and extension, as well as in pronation and supination, can help provide a better view of the joint. An example is shown in Figure 30.

Wrist Joint

The trocar is introduced into the dorsal aspect of the wrist joint, whether at a point on the ulnar side of the extensor pollicis longus tendon or at a point between the lunate and radius (Fig. 31). The latter method was called the lateral approach by Burman.

In making the trocar puncture, the extensor pollicis longus tendon should be carefully palpated to avoid injury to the tendon. In arthroscopy of a rheumatoid wrist joint, the lateral approach is recommended instead of the medial approach, as the tendon here has often become fragile.

The wrist is kept in a slightly dorsiflexed position while the trocar puncture is made. The area observed is restricted to the dorsal portion of the radionavicular and scaphoulnar

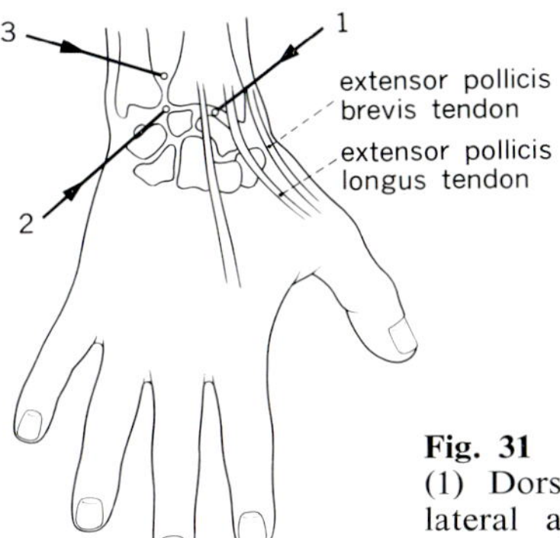

Fig. 31 Approach to the wrist joint. (1) Dorsal medial approach. (2) Dorsal lateral approach. (3) Approach to the distal radioulnar joint.

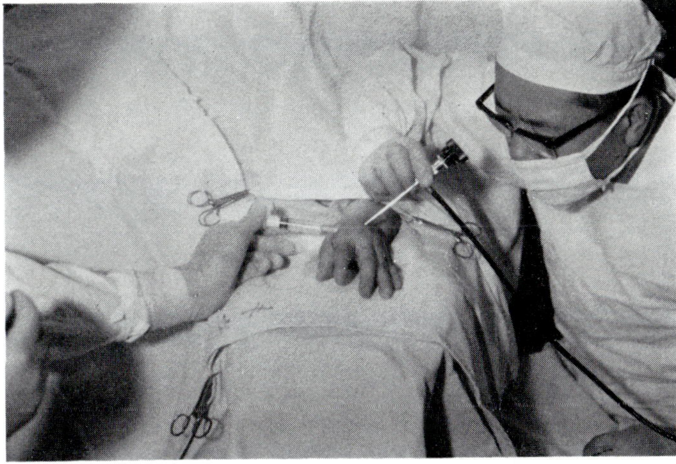

Fig. 32 Arthroscopy of the metacarpophalangeal joint.

joints. The authors prefer the lateral approach and the use of a fore-oblique viewing scope. A widened view may be obtained by repeated use of an obturator in moving the scope in joint.

Distal Radioulnar Joint

Normally, this joint is quite narrow, rendering arthroscopic visualization rather limited. A swollen arthritic joint, however, often permits observation of the joint cavity filled with inflammatory villi. The trocar is introduced into the joint from a slightly proximal and dorsal aspect.

Metacarpophalangeal Joint

The joint is entered in the area between the common extensor tendon and the collateral ligament (Figs. 32 and 33). In order to observe the joint cavity, traction must be exerted on the finger and considerable distension with normal saline is necessary.

Proximal and Distal Interphalangeal Joints

Arthroscopy of the proximal and distal interphalangeal joints is possible only when they are quite swollen. The technique employed is similar to that used in arthroscopy of the metacarpophalangeal joint.

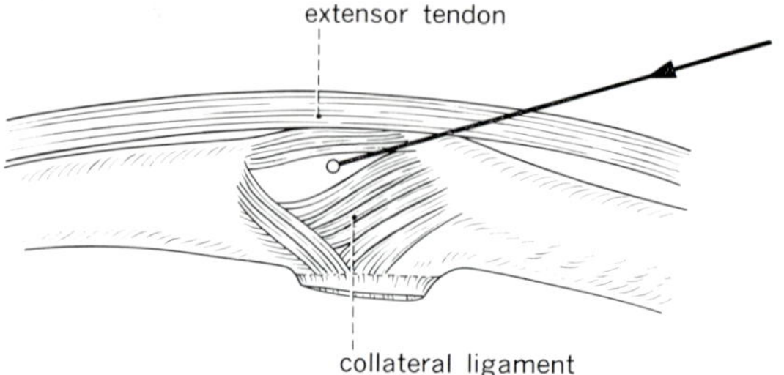

Fig. 33 Approach to the metacarpophalangeal joint.

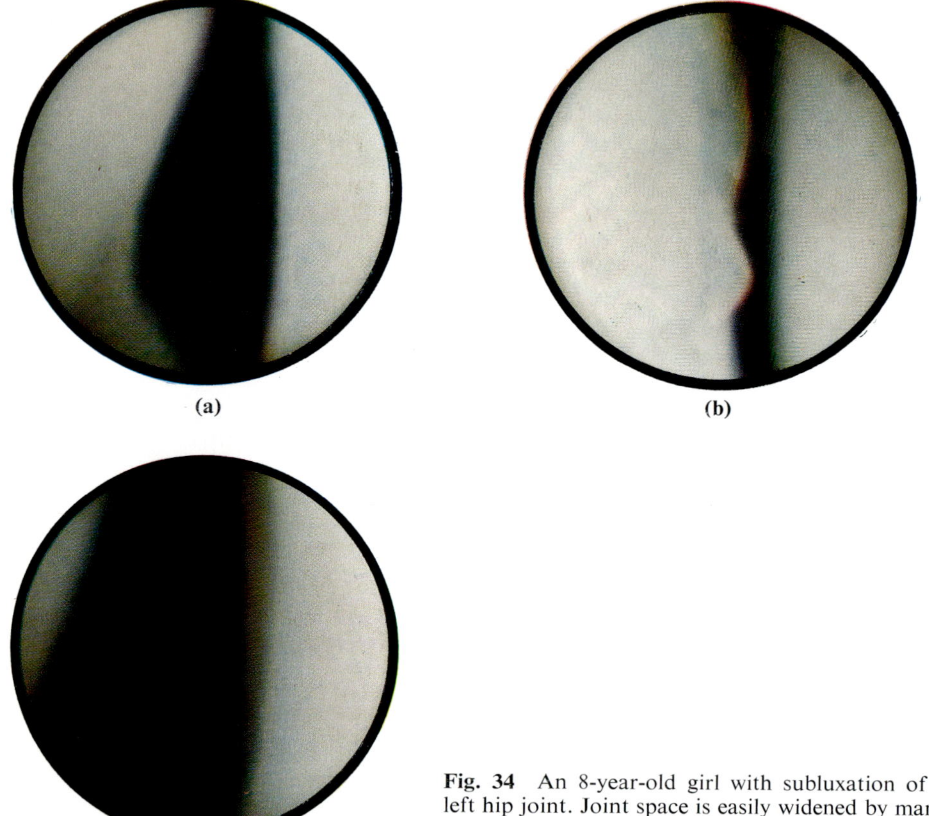

Fig. 34 An 8-year-old girl with subluxation of the left hip joint. Joint space is easily widened by manual traction.

Hip Joint

The anterior pertrochanteric approach has been found to be satisfactory. The puncture is carried out under control of a roentgen image. The joint is maintained in external rotation. Although visualization of the acetablum is restricted, a part of the extraacetabular part of the femoral head and the intraarticular part of the neck of the femur are visible.

Child's Hip Joint

In a child's hip joint—especially in a dislocated hip joint—arthroscopy is much easier than with adult hip joints. Manual traction is usually effective in distracting the head from its socket (Fig. 34). Such manual traction is not effective in the case of adult hip joint.

Observation is made with rotation, abduction, flexion, and traction. In some cases, the limbus, the fovea, and a part of the ligamentum capitis femoris can also be seen. Observation should be performed by gentle movement of the scope and the femoral head while viewing the cartilaginous surface very closely and obtaining a very narrow field of vision.

Ankle Joint

The No. 24-A and No. 24-B scopes are used for arthroscopy of the ankle joint. A clinical study found that hydrostatic pressure between 70 mmHg and 190 mmHg was necessary to obtain a clear view of the ankle joint. Although the anteromedial and anterolateral routes (Fig. 35) are commonly used, a posterior approach (Fig. 36) that avoids the Achilles tendon and posterior neurovascular bundle can sometimes be helpful. The anterior joint space and the talomalleolar joint can be observed by the anterior approach. Examples are shown in Figure 37.

Metatarsophalangeal Joint and Interphalangeal Joint

The articulation between the hallux and its metatarsal is entered at a point either lateral or medial to the extensor tendon. As this joint is extremely difficult to open with manual traction, a 2.0-mm outside diameter sheath must be used.

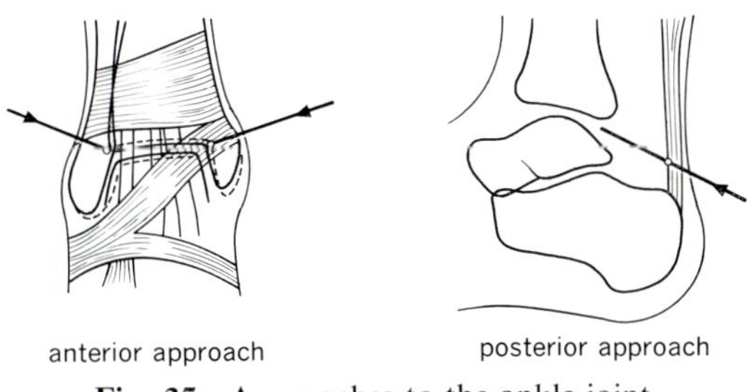

Fig. 35 Approaches to the ankle joint.

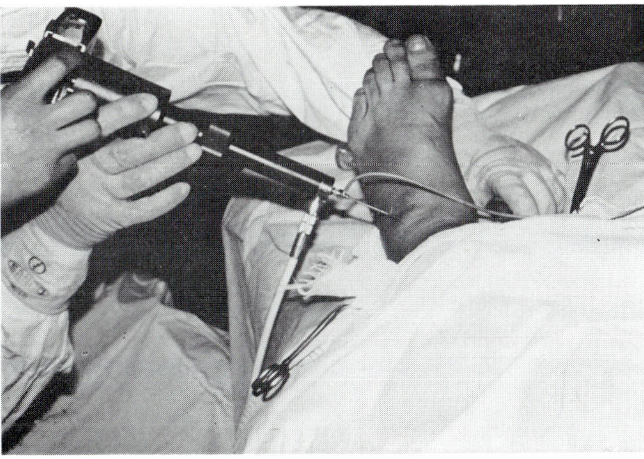

Fig. 36 Anterior lateral approach to the ankle joint.

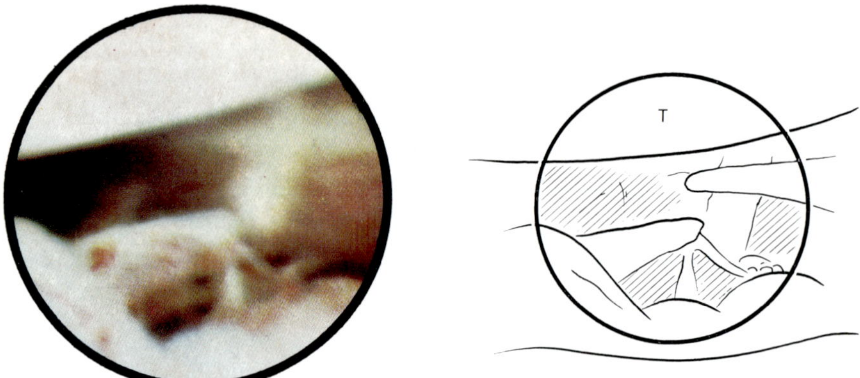

Fig. 37 A 28-year-old woman with rheumatoid arthritis of the right ankle joint. Necrotic villi are seen. (T) Tibia.

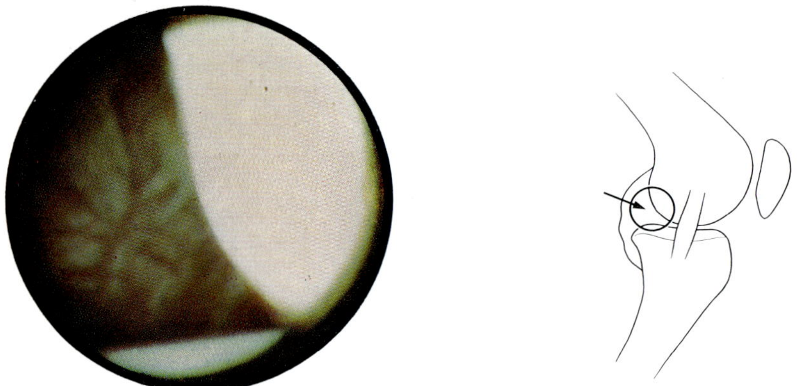

Fig. 38 View of posterior part of the medial meniscus, medial posterior approach.

In the other metatarsophalangeal joints, manual traction is effective for widening the joint space.

Knee Joint

The No. 24 arthroscope is not suitable for general diagnostic purposes in the knee joint. The No. 24 is used for observation of the posterior part of the medial meniscus by posterior medial approach (Fig. 38). The posteromedial puncture is easy when the knee is sufficiently distended with normal saline, flexed to 60°, and in varus position. For observation of the undersurface of the meniscus, the posterior cruciate ligament, etc., the No. 24 should be used in tandem with the No. 21 and a probe or an intraarticular retractor.

Bursas and Tendon Sheaths

The No. 24 arthroscope can be used for swollen bursas and tendon sheaths.

PUNCH BIOPSY

In arthroscopy of small joints with the No. 24, punch biopsy is a half-blind procedure in most cases. After careful inspection, the object of biopsy is selected and the scope is directed to the object. Then the scope is gently withdrawn and the biopsy punch is introduced through the same sheath for blind punch biopsy. This method may be called a half-blind punch biopsy. Because the punch (Fig. 39) and consequently the specimens taken are extremely small, care must be taken to collect a sufficient number of specimens.

Punch biopsy under arthroscopic control is performed through a separate sheath introduced into the joint and brought into the field of vision. This is possible in selected cases by two approaches. For example, it is possible with anteromedial and anterolateral approaches in the ankle joint, dorsoradial and dorsoulnar approaches in the wrist joint, and posteroradial and posteroulnar approaches in the elbow joint.

Figure 40 shows punch biopsy under No. 24-A arthroscopic visualization.

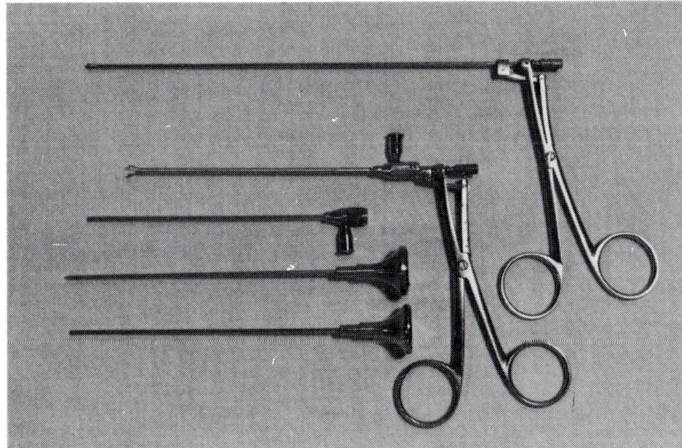

Fig. 39 Biopsy punches.

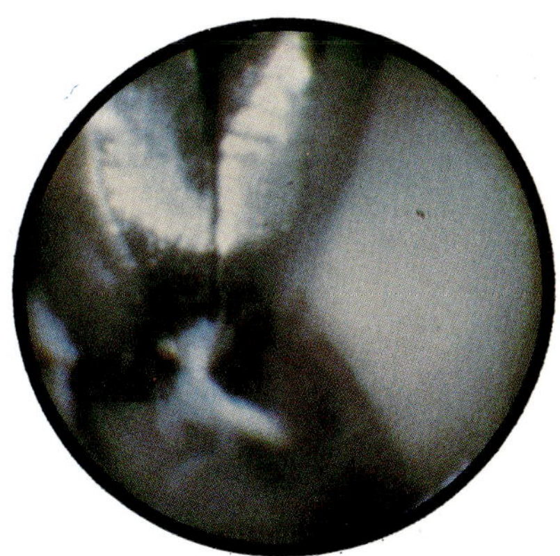

Fig. 40 Punch biopsy under No. 24-A arthroscopic visualization of the right elbow joint in a case of rheumatoid arthritis in a 77-year-old woman.

SURGERY UNDER ARTHROSCOPIC CONTROL

Generally speaking, arthroscopic surgery in small joints is at present a difficult procedure. Manipulation of surgical instruments under arthroscopic control is more difficult than manipulation of a biopsy punch.

Of course there are cases in which removal of loose bodies in the shoulder, elbow, or ankle joint is achieved under arthroscopy. In most cases, however, removal of loose bodies in the joint is performed blindly through a minimum incision according to a plan made by careful arthroscopic examination. Arthroscopic synovectomy in rheumatoid joints and arthroscopic drilling in osteochondritis dissecans have also been performed.

In the near future, marked progress is expected in the field of arthroscopic surgery on small joints, as has been achieved in the field of arthroscopic knee surgery.

PHOTOGRAPHY AND COLOR TV

Photographs may be taken through the No. 24 by setting the light source (150 W) at sufficient brightness. Progress in color film, camera, and illumination has permitted satisfactory photographic recording of the interior view of small joints. The authors use Ektachrome (EA) (ASA 400), with an exposure time of one-fifteenth to one-eighth second.

Figures 41 through 44 are photographs taken by one of the authors (K. I.).

Popularization of arthroscopy was delayed by the necessity for one-to-one teaching. To overcome this difficulty, the development of a video system available not only for knee joint arthroscopy but also for small joint arthroscopy was essential. However, it was very difficult to produce a video system sensitive enough to obtain clear video images through the small arthroscope.

In 1978, Watanabe and Takeda developed a color video system of high-sensitivity and high-quality image for arthroscopy, in cooperation with the Technical Institute of NHK (Japan Broadcasting Association). It was available not only for knee joint arthroscopy, but also for small joint arthroscopy (Fig. 45).

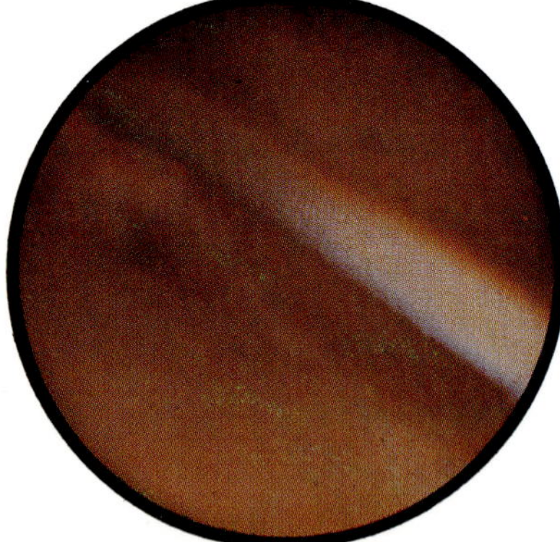

Fig. 41 A 17-year-old girl with recurrent dislocation of the left shoulder joint, posterior approach. (Middle) Biceps longus tendon, reduced in thickness. (Below) Humeral head.

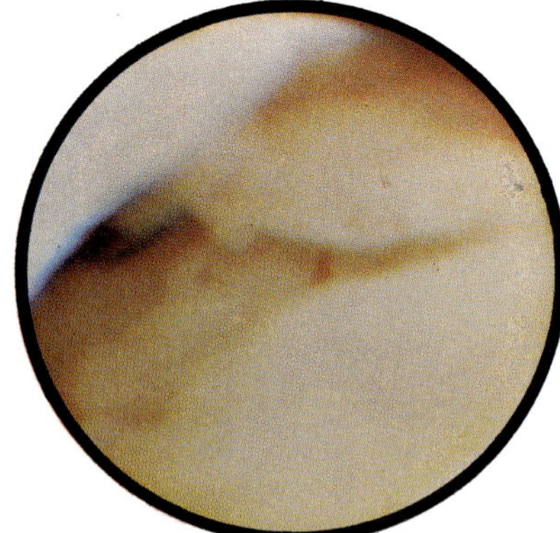

Fig. 42 A 40-year-old man with Kienböck's disease, left wrist joint. (Left above) Radius. (Right) Lunatum. The lunate bone looks yellow. Fracture is also seen.

Subsequently, a smaller color TV called Circon was developed in the United States and popularized. Circon has been used in many hospitals in Japan. Recently, smaller TV cameras were manufactured also in Japan by Sony and Olympus. The Olympus TV camera weighs 280 g (Fig. 46). More recently, a semiconductor TV camera was developed by Stryker Company of the United States and Shinko Optical Company in Japan, respectively. The latter is the maker of the Watanabe No. 21 arthroscope. Shinko's semiconductor camera (Fig. 47) weighs only 260 g and is of high sensitivity and high quality. It can also be used in small joint arthroscopy with Selfoscope.

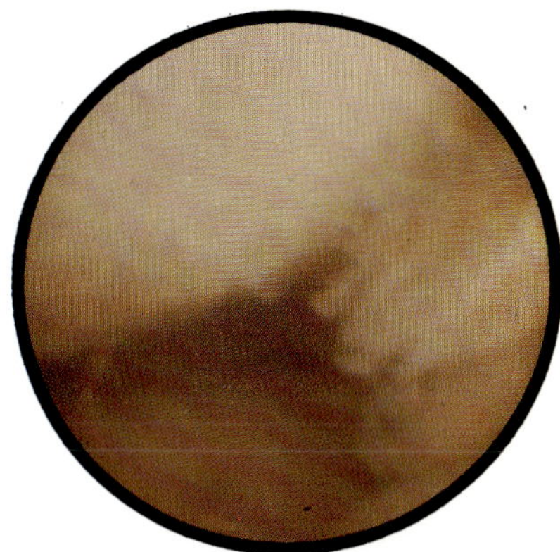

Fig. 43 A 17-year-old girl with rupture of a collateral ligament, proximal interphalangeal joint of the right index finger. (Top) Middle phalanx. (Below) Basic phalanx. On the right, ruptured and invaginated collateral ligament is seen.

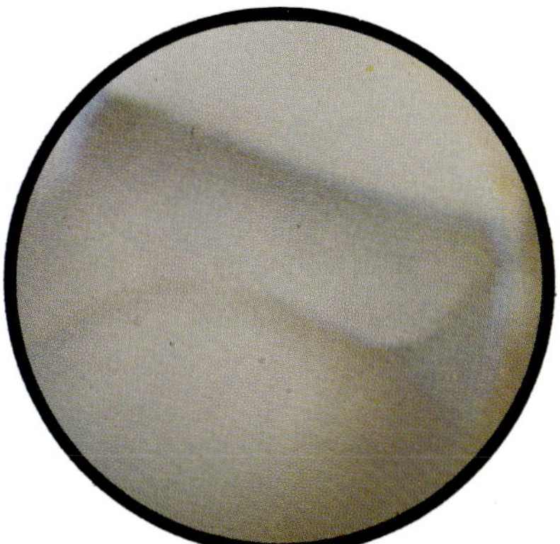

Fig. 44 An 18-year-old boy, left ankle joint. Lateral anterior approach. (Top) Tibia. (Below) Talus. A cartilage-like plica is seen in the middle part.

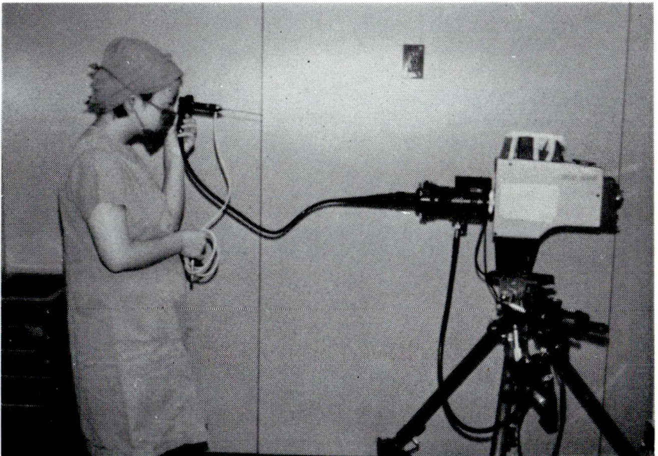

Fig. 45 Color video system of high sensitivity and high quality.

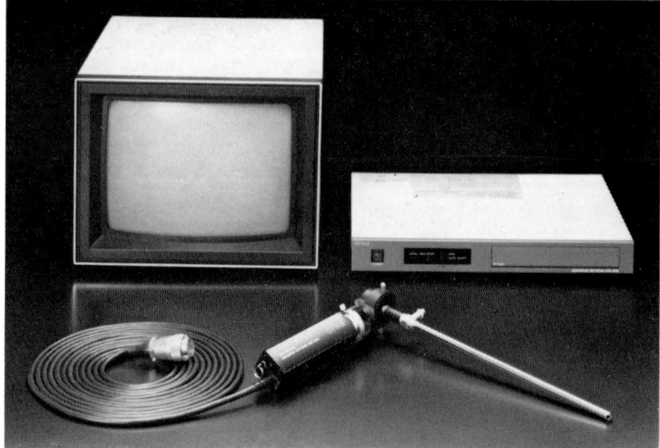

Fig. 46 A TV system for endoscopic observation including arthroscopy, TV adaptor, TV camera, and camera-control unit (Olympus Optical, Tokyo).

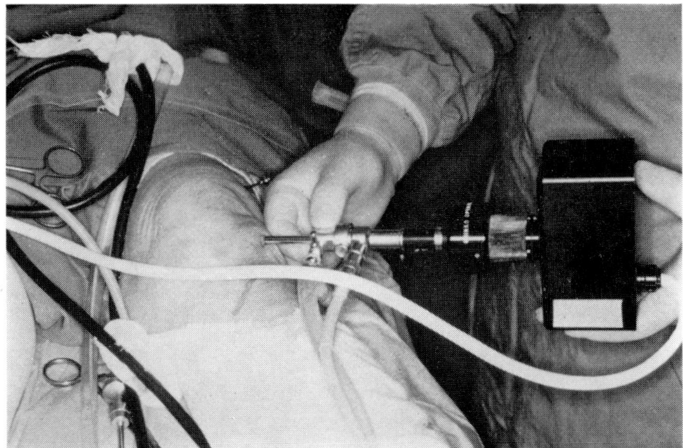

Fig. 47 The practice of arthroscopy with a new TV camera recently developed by Shinko Optical, Tokyo.

2

Recording of Small Joint Arthroscopy

ARTHROSCOPIC PHOTOGRAPHY

Currently, the Watanabe No. 24 arthroscope (Selfoscope) is the most useful instrument for arthroscopic observation and photography of small joints. The fore-oblique viewing arthroscope is especially suitable because of its 41° visual field and the possibility of obtaining a 52° visual field by rotating the scope within the outer sheath.

The basic precautions for arthroscopic photography of small joints are similar to those for the knee joint when using the No. 21 arthroscope.

The following section describes specific techniques for small joint arthroscopic photography with the No. 24 arthroscope.

Normal saline is introduced into the joint cavity under pressure with either a syringe or irrigator for arthroscopic observation. When the pressure of the joint cavity is greatly increased, the color of synovial membrane becomes pale. This paling tends to reflect the illumination and allows use of faster camera shutter speeds.

For the No. 24 in particular, the following cautions are noted.

The light guide in the No. 24 arthroscope is small, thus illumination decreases rapidly with the distance of the arthroscope from the viewed object. The proper exposure time for objects situated at different distances from the lens will differ, even though they may be in the same visual field. Care must be taken in this respect.

The visual field is apt to be obscured by synovial villi and fibrillation of articular cartilage contacting the object lens of the arthroscope in the narrow cavity of the small joint. Should this occur, draw the arthroscope back into the sheath several millimeters so that there is a small space in front of the tip of the scope which will allow for observation and photography.

Camera

A 35-mm single-lens reflex camera, which allows the operator to photograph what is directly observed through the viewfinder, is usually used for arthroscopic photography of small joints. For the No. 24 arthroscope, the Olympus OM-1 camera is standard, though others may suffice. The Olympus OM series cameras have a mounting attachment for the No. 24. For other manufacturers' cameras, mounting attachments must be ordered. The manual exposure meter on the Olympus OM-1 cannot be used because the exposure setting register at the left side of the viewfinder cannot be read, as only light from the convex lens at the center of the focusing screen is seen. Therefore proper exposure time must be determined either through an automatic exposure system or from an exposure meter adapted from that used for microscopes.

The Olympus OM-2 and OM-10 are equipped with automatic exposure systems that give fairly good exposures, relieving the operator of having to continually adjust the shutter speed. Regretfully, repeated sterilization in formalin gas adversely affects these automatic exposure systems.

Motor drive unit: One problem that can occur during arthroscopic photography of small joints is bending of the arthroscope's stainless steel tube, which may happen during observation or film winding. Distortion of the normally spherical visual field is an indication of this and a warning that the arthroscope may break. Thus the operator must be careful not to bend the tube of the arthroscope while observing, and photography should not be attempted if the visual field becomes very distorted. A motor drive for the OM series is available from Olympus and allows the operator to wind the film quickly and smoothly without taking his eye from the viewfinder. The disadvantage of the motor drive is that it is relatively heavy and bulky.

Camera adaptor: An adaptor interfaces between the arthroscope and camera. In addition to the mechanical linkage, the adaptor also reduces the arthroscope's wide field of vision and focuses the image on the camera's focal plane. The adaptor does not have an aperture control mechanism, so exposure is determined entirely by shutter speed.

The diameter of the arthroscopic photogram is determined by the lens in the adaptor. Standard photograms have diameters of about 1.0 cm. With the use of enlarging links such as the Olympus Teleconverter 2X-A, the Kenko Teleplus MC 7 and MC 4, etc., larger diameters are possible.

Large-diameter photograms require greater illumination. This may be accomplished by using slow shutter speeds, but at speeds slower than one-quarter second, blurring due to camera shake occurs. To avoid speeds slower than one-quarter second, a high-power illumination source may be necessary.

Alternately, 1-cm diameter photograms may be enlarged.

Proper Exposure

Color slide film has a narrower latitude than color negative film, so its exposure time is the more critical.

Also, exposure differs by subject; for example, the whitish surface of cartilage versus the reddish surface or synovial membrane. The exposure for each shot must be determined independently of the previous one.

For the No. 24 arthroscope, proper exposure is determined by the following factors:

Without electronic flash—
- Shutter speed
- Intensity of illumination

With electronic flash—
- Duration of flash

Shutter speed: The most common speeds are one-quarter, one-eighth, and one-fifteenth, with one-eighth second being the lower limit for sharpness. Faster shutter speeds are desirable to avoid blurring due to camera shake. For poorly illuminated shots where a shutter speed slower than one-quarter second is indicated, it is preferable to have the developing laboratory specially process the film to effectively double the film's speed.

Cameras with aperture-preference automatic exposure systems allow fairly good photograms and require only that the operator focuses the image properly. However, there is a tendency toward overexposure because of the strong reflection from the glossy, white surface of the cartilage, which results in the fine contour of fibrillation of articular cartilage becoming vague.

An autoexposure compensation system, such as on the Olympus OM-2, can correct this tendency by varying the exposure up to two f-stops.

Intensity of the light source: At present, the author considers a xenon short-arc lamp to be the best illumination source for the No. 24 arthroscope. The author's hospital usually uses light sources manufactured by either Machida or Olympus that have 500-W xenon short-arc lamps.

The subject is usually illuminated at the maximum intensity possible to allow fast shutter speeds. However, too bright illumination source will "wash out" the subject, fading the natural colors of the tissue. Therefore, the intensity of light within the visual field must be controlled during observation.

The Olympus CLX-F (Table 6) is equipped with through-the-lens autoexposure using an electronic flash, which is suitable for the various gastrofiberscopes and endoscopes equipped with light sensors. Regretfully, these cannot be used with the No. 24, which is too slender to fit a light sensor.

Olympus has recently introduced two accessories for the No. 24: the Olympus SC16-3R, a small camera for 16-mm film; and the SM-EFR, an adaptor equipped with an electronic-flash sensor that can interface between the arthroscope and OM-1 or OM-2 cameras (See Electronic flash section).

Electronic flash: In systems equipped with an electronic flash, proper exposure is determined by controlling the duration of the flash. An electronic flash can produce a stronger illumination than the maximum possible for visual observation, thus allowing proper exposure of distant subjects.

The SC16–3R camera is smaller than the OM series cameras, and its light weight is an advantage. It is equipped with a sensor to control the electronic flash system. It uses 16-mm film, the photograms of which must be enlarged to 35-mm format. The image formed by the SC16–3R is sufficiently sharp for this purpose.

The SM-EFR (EE adaptor for OM-1 and OM-2) is an adaptor equipped with an electronic-flash sensor that interfaces between the No. 24 and OM-1 or OM-2.

Both the SC16-3R and the SM-EFR can be used with the illumination sources manufactured by Olympus (Table 6).

Generally, when an electronic flash is used with a focalplane-shutter camera, the shutter speed should be slower than one-sixtieth second to avoid the shutter curtain cutting off the exposure, resulting in a portion of the photogram being underexposed. For the CLX-F, shutter speed should be slower than one-eighth second, as stipulated by the manufacturer.

One problem with using an electronic flash in small joint arthroscopy is excessive illumination. In taking photographs in the small joints where the space is very narrow the flash

Table 6 Illumination sources by Olympus Optical

	CLE-F	CLS-F	CLX-F
Illumination	150-W halogen lamp	150-W xenon short-arc lamp (350 VA)	500-W xenon short-arc lamp (1,000 VA)
Flash	Xenon flash lamp	Xenon flash lamp (1,000 VA)	Xenon short-arc lamp (5,000 VA)
Automatic exposure	Synchronized shutter speeds slower than one-sixtieth second	Synchronized shutter speeds slower than one-eighth second	Synchronized shutter speeds slower than one-eighth second

may bring too much halation of the cartilage. As electronic-flash sensors are developed and put into use, electronic-flash systems will come into general use in small joint arthroscopy. Close-up shots of synovial tissue and microscopically enlarged stop-action shots of synovial villi using very fast shutter speeds will become possible, leading to new fields of arthroscopic study.

Exposure Meter

As mentioned above, the OM-1's built-in exposure meter cannot be used for arthroscopic photograms. As relying on the operator's subjective estimates will likely lead to error, some means of measuring the amount of light reaching the film must be devised. Unfortunately, Olympus does not manufacture an exposure meter designed specifically for arthroscopic use. However, a metering system has been adapted from one designed for microscopes. The Olympus EMM-6 photomicrographic exposure meter can be fitted with a sensor viewfinder that interfaces with the OM series cameras and that measures the intensity of light at the center of the focusing screen (Figs. 48–50). It is sterilized in formalin gas.

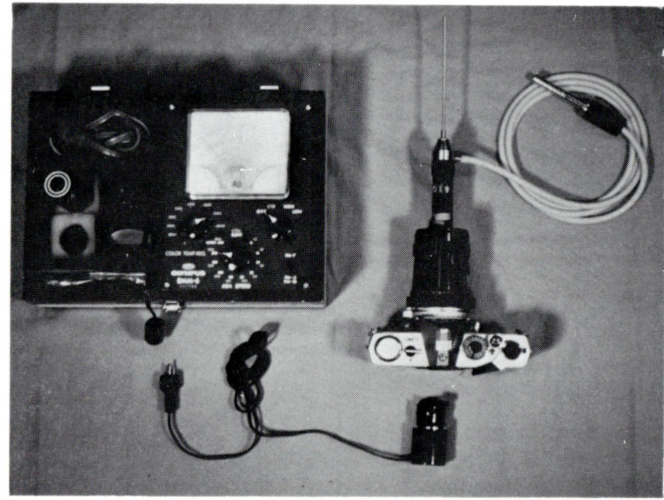

Fig. 48

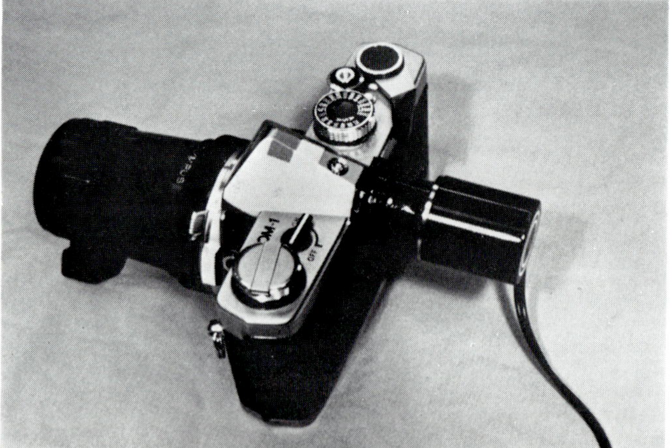

Fig. 49

Figs. 48, 49 An exposure meter, adapted from one made for microscopes, is fitted to the center of the viewfinder of the camera.

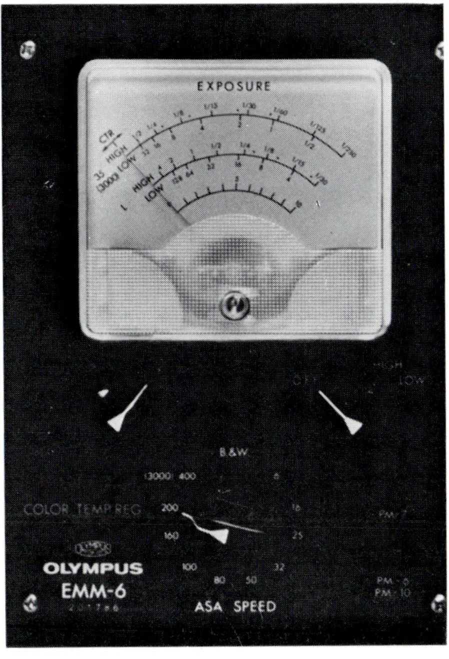

Fig. 50 Exposure monitor with ASA-select knob and meter dial set to shutter speed. The shutter speed of the proper exposure condition can be easily determined even if the arthroscopist wants to increase the effective speed of the film to two times that of the ASA.

Film

For arthroscopy, 35-mm film is most often used. It is capable of being projected during meetings and conferences. Tungsten film is used with the halogen lamp, which is the more portable of the light sources, while daylight film is used with the xenon lamp, which is the higher power light source. Daylight film is also used with the electronic flash. The author usually shoots Kodak Ektachrome 160 (ET) (ASA 160) with a tungsten lamp and Kodak Ektachrome 400 (EL) (ASA 400) with a xenon lamp.

The Kodak Ektachrome 400 (daylight) (EL) is the most sensitive film available on the general market and can be processed within several hours, if necessary. Furthermore, the film speed can be effectively doubled to ASA 800 by special processing. Thus should an unacceptably slow shutter speed of one-half second be indicated, the shutter speed can still be set at an acceptable speed of one-quarter second and the film specially processed to ASA 800.

The film used should be compatible with the color temperature of the light source. Tungsten film takes on a blue hue if used with a xenon lamp, and daylight film turns red-yellow with a halogen lamp.

If the film has been mistakenly exposed with the wrong light source, the processing laboratory may be able to correct the color by use of a filter (Figs. 51 and 52). It is best in such circumstances to provide the laboratory with a sample of properly exposed film to use as a reference.

If an incompatible film must be used, perhaps because the higher speed daylight film must be used with a halogen lamp, a color-correction filter may be used when photographing. Usually the filter is placed on top of the adaptor, though it could be inserted anywhere along the light system. The color-correction filters made by Fuji Film are of washable acetate and are thus superior to Kodak's gelatin filters for arthroscopic use.

Care and storage of film: All film must be protected from moisture and high tempe-

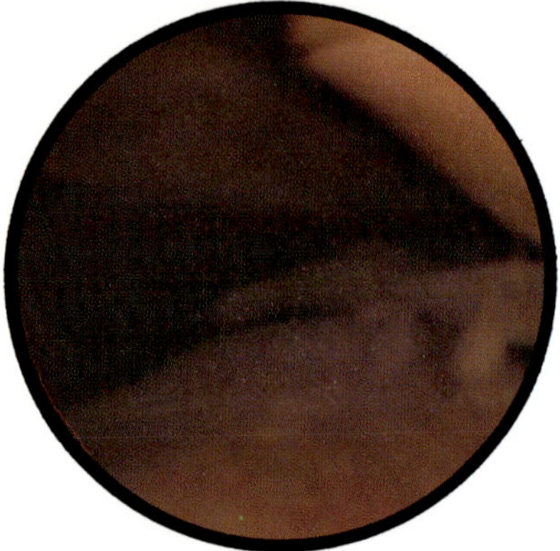
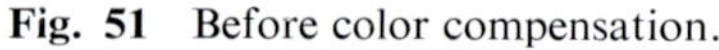

Fig. 51 Before color compensation.

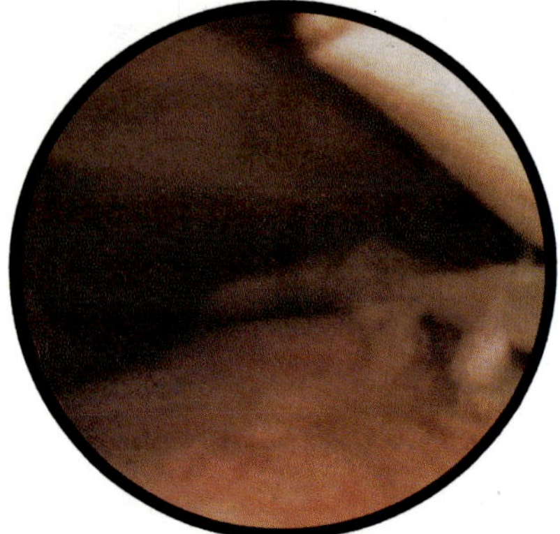

Fig. 52 After color compensation.

rature. Unexposed film must be used before the end of its shelf life and should be stored in a refrigerator. Film should be removed from the refrigerator about one hour before use. Developed film should be stored in a cool, dark place, preferably with desiccants, to minimize color fading.

Miscellaneous Points

The first frame of each roll of film should include the date, patient name, joint name, side (right or left), approach, and so on written on the data paper. This will greatly aid in arranging the developed film later.

Paper and pencils, sterilized in formalin gas, should be prepared. A sketch of the findings accompanied with a brief description will help in orienting the photograms later. Also, sketches record more information than operation reports.

The camera must be sterilized in formalin gas. It is operated by the surgeon.

Good photograms require a clear visual field. When normal saline is introduced into the joint to clear the visual field, it is most effective to inject it directly through the trocar.

Synovial villi and fibrillation of articular cartilage are best photographed after the flow of normal saline has been stopped.

It is important to establish a constant orientation for the frames, i.e., the bottom always running parallel to the long axis of the extremity. This will aid in understanding and evaluation, especially for the No. 24 arthroscope, which has a narrower visual field than the No. 21.

COLOR TV MONITORING

Color TV systems have become indispensable for arthroscopic surgery. The arthroscopic image on the TV screen permits operating staff to work together during arthroscopic surgery, and lets nurses help the surgeon efficiently. By use of a color TV system and a mock-up, training of beginning surgeons and students is more immediate and efficient.

Diagnostic as well as operative arthroscopy can easily be videotaped for permanent record. The videotape is protected in a sturdy plastic videocassette case. The safety cap at the bottom of videocassette case prevents accidental overlapping of recordings or erasing of recorded arthroscopic images.

At present, there are three different types of the video recording systems. They are classified according to the width of the videotape: one inch, one-half inch, and three-quarter inch.

The one-inch tape is commonly used by specialists. This tape is the best quality and the most expensive among the three. The one-half inch tape, the smallest size tape, is used with the common home video system and costs the least of the three types. The three-quarter inch tape has sufficient quality for arthroscopic recording. Many problems have arisen in editing videocassette tapes of different sizes, and especially in interchanging images among different color signal systems. There are three different color signal systems in the world: PAL and SECAM in Europe, and $NTSC_{4.43}$ in the United States and Japan. The most prevailing video system in the world today is the U-matic system with three-quarter inch video cassette tapes. This size video-cassette tape is the best for arthroscopy recording, editing, and tape-to-tape editing.

Development of a clinical arthroscopic TV system for the knee joint was started by John McGinty in 1975. In 1976, Masaki Watanabe and Sakae Takeda attempted development of a new color TV system suitable not only for knee joint arthroscopy, but also for small joint arthroscopy. The light guide in the Watanabe No. 24 and other thin arthroscopes for small joints is small; thus illumination decreases rapidly with the distance of the arthroscope from the object, necessitating a more sensitive color TV camera. In 1978, Watanabe succeeded in developing the highly sensitive high-quality color TV system. By the use of this system good arthroscopic video images of various small joints could be achieved. Since 1980, the commercial Hitachi (Tokyo) high-sensitivity color TV camera system has been in use in the author's hospital (See Fig. 45). It is equipped with a zoom lens, which permits selection of ideal image size. The lecture scope, which is of high quality and is chemical inert in the disinfecting gas, is connected to the tip of the zoom lens and to the arthroscope. The flexible lecture scope allows the surgeon free movement of the arthroscope.

Since the development of a microvideo camera by Circon Corporation in the United States, color TV video systems have been popularized throughout the world.

The Sony and Olympus companies in Japan have also offered their own smaller color TV camera systems (See Fig. 46).

Recently, solid-state microelectric circuitry has been applied to new color TV camera systems. Solid-state color TV camera systems offer many practical advancements over ordinary vidicon cameras. They have resolved the problems of image burn, ghosting, flaring, flashing, and geometric distortion, that were unavoidable with conventional vidicon cameras. Solid-state sensors work out a fine color balance between dark areas and bright white areas, and have high sensitivity. As a result, it is possible to get fine, color-balanced arthroscopic images on the monitor. Also, solid-state sensors have been used to develope a tiny, lightweight, immersible arthroscopic color TV camera. The newest color TV cameras have been commercially produced by Circon (Santa Barbara, Calif.), Medical Dynamic (Englewood, Colorado), Shinko Optical (Tokyo) (See Fig. 47), and Storz (Tuttlingen, West Germany), Stryker (Kalamazoo, Mich.), Wolf (Rosemont, Illinois). Even now development of color TV systems for arthroscopy is a growing field.

II

CLINICAL APPLICATIONS

3

Clinical Applications of the No. 24 Arthroscope

Clinical application of arthroscopy of joints other than the knee has at last been made possible with the 1.7-mm diameter Watanabe No. 24 arthroscope (Selfoscope).

Arthroscopy of small joints differs from knee arthroscopy in that it is impossible to observe most of the whole joint cavity through one puncture. In arthroscopy of small joints, identification of intraarticular structures is difficult because the joint cavity is narrow and the visual field is limited. Clinical visualization of small joints therefore demands an accurate knowledge of the gross anatomy and pathology of these joints.

As reported by the author in the *Atlas of Arthroscopy, 3rd edition* (Watanabe et al. 1978, p. 28), the No. 24 arthroscope was tested on over 400 joints other than the knee in the period from January 1970 to March 1975.

From April, 1975 until March 31, 1982, approximately 500 joints other than the knee were studied by arthroscopy in Tokyo Teishin Hospital (Table 7).

As shown in Table 7, about one third of the arthroscopy cases are of rheumatoid arthritis. In active arthritic joints, the joint cavity is filled with proliferated villi and necrotic masses, so it is difficult to identify other joint structures such as cartilaginous surfaces and ligaments. However, the finding of proliferated villi and necrotic masses in itself can be said to be characteristic of rheumatoid joints.

BIOPSY

Biopsy specimens taken by the No. 24 biopsy punch are very small, and occasionally they are too small for disease diagnosis. However, when there is a proliferation of villi in the joint, moving the tip of the sheath gradually can facilitate multiple punch biopsies and a sufficient number of specimens can be obtained (Fig. 53).

DISEASES DETECTED BY THE NO. 24 ARTHROSCOPE

Occasionally, correct diagnosis of osteochondral fracture, osteochondritis dissecans, and loose bodies can be made first by arthroscopy. Arthroscopy is also useful in judging pathological findings of intraarticular tendon such as biceps brachii tendon in the shoulder joint, some changes of the rotator cuff, or chondral fracture of the child's elbow joint (Watanabe et al. 1978, p. 139). Chondral fracture in the sprained ankle joint is occasionally detected by arthroscopy.

Among joints other than the knee, the adult hip joint is most difficult to visualize

Table 7 Clinical cases, Tokyo Teishin Hospital, joints other than knee examined with the No. 24 arthroscope (April 1, 1975 to March 31, 1982)

Joint examined	Number	Rheumatoid arthritis	Gouty arthritis	Other arthritides	Osteo-arthritis	Fracture	Other diagnosis (number)
Temporomandibular joint	3						Derangement (3)
Sternoclavicular joint	1			1			
Shoulder joint	72	20		4		2	Recurrent dislocation (3), tendon rupture (6), loose bodies of unknown origin (2), contracture (6), others (29)
Elbow joint	122	48	1	5	11	26	Dislocation (3), osteochondritis dissecans (8), osteochondromatosis (1), chondrocalcinosis (1), loose bodies of unknown origin (1), hemarthrosis (1), flail joint (1), others (15)
Wrist joint (including distal radioulnar joint)	38	22		4		10	Lunatomalacia (1), others (1)
First carpometacarpal joint	1			1			
Metacarpophalangeal joint	30	27	1				Locking of sesamoid bones (2)
Interphalangeal and proximal interphalangeal joint	4	2	2				
Distal interphalangeal joint	1			1			
Hip joint (adult)	43	8		1	19	8	Aseptic necrosis (4), loose bodies (2), exostosis (1), congenital dislocation (8), Perthes' disease (3), slipped proximal femoral epiphysis (1)
Hip joint (child's)	12						
Ankle joint	163	32	3	19	12	29	Sprain (38), osteochondritis dissecans (4), aseptic necrosis (1), osteochondromatosis (1), loose bodies of unknown origin (3), extracapsular ectopic ossification (2), others (19)
Metatarsophalangeal joint	12	10	2				
Total	502	169	9	36	42	75	171

Also examined:
tendon sheath of extensor digitorum communis muscle (tendon rupture) 1; calcaneal tendon 17 (rupture 15, tumor 2); bursa (bursitis) 7; soft-tissue tumor 1

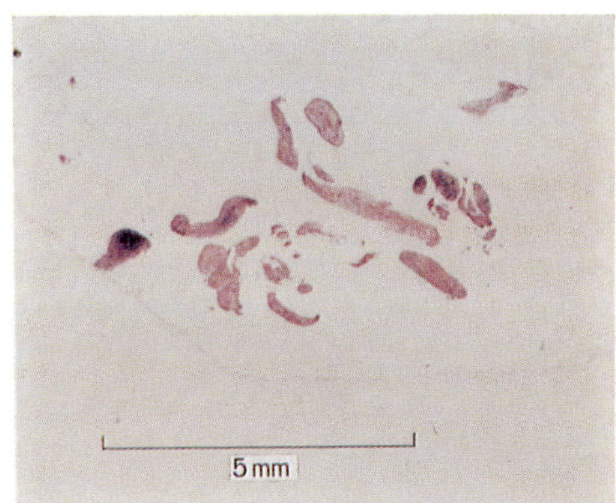

Fig. 53 Biopsy specimen of the synovium taken by No. 24 biopsy punch. Rheumatoid arthritis, elbow joint. Hematoxylin-eosin stain (×6).

through the arthroscope. As the joint is situated deep within the body, it is difficult to move the tip of the scope in a single approach. Moreover, the central areas of the femoral head and acetabulum are in close contact. In the child's hip joint, especially in a dislocated hip joint, arthroscopy is much easier and more useful than that in the adult hip joint.

In a case of old medial malleolar fracture, arthroscopy prior to open reduction was useful for learning the condition of displacement of the articular surface and for planning the operation.

THERAPEUTIC EFFECT

In rheumatoid arthritis and other arthritides, joint effusion and pain frequently subside for several weeks after arthroscopy. This is believed to be the effect of joint perfusion with normal saline for one-half to one hour's duration (Watanabe, 1950; Watanabe and Nagatsuka, 1969; Sakakibara, 1973). Therapeutic effect of joint perfusion, likely caused by removal of some pathological substances in the joint, is now under investigation.

In the frozen shoulder and other joint contractures, arthroscopy is effective in improving the range of motion and in relieving pain (Conti, 1979).

In the elbow, ankle, and other joints, loose bodies can be located exactly by arthroscopy, and can then be removed through a small incision. The period of immobilization of the joint is thus reduced.

Details of clinical applications of arthroscopy in each joint are discussed in Chapters 5 through 11.

4

Arthroscopy of the Shoulder Joint

ARTHROSCOPIC ANATOMY OF THE SHOULDER JOINT

The shoulder joint is a spheroid joint consisting of the humeral head and the glenoid cavity of the scapula. The glenoid cavity is surrounded with a limbus (labrum glenoidale) at the rim, but the humeral head is bigger than the cavity so that the acromion, the coracoid process, and the coracoacromial ligament support the joint as a ligamentous dome. The outside of the capsule has a fibrous connection with the coracohumeral ligament and the supraspinatus, infraspinatus, teres minor, and subscapularis muscle tendons around the capsule. From the tendons of these muscles, fibrous tissue attaches to the outer side of the capsule for reinforcement. These four tendons are called the rotator cuff. The inferior portion of the capsule is thin, but the other portions are thick.

The intraarticular cavity is divided into four cavities—the superior, inferior, anterior, and posterior—and the glenohumeral joint space. In the cavity there are the glenoid cavity of the scapular bone; the limbus; the humeral head; the long head of the brachial biceps tendon; the superior, middle, and inferior glenohumeral ligaments; and synovial villi (Fig. 54). The long head lies embedded in the posterosuperior portion of the glenoid process. The superior and middle glenohumeral ligaments begin from the anterosuperior portion of the glenoid process, and the inferior glenohumeral ligament begins from the middle portion of the anterior rim. In front of the attachment of the superior glenohumeral ligament there is a small anterior recess (Fig. 55). The subscapular bursa opens inferiorly in half of all cases. Variations in the glenohumeral ligament can occasionally be seen. Some variations are a cord- or fold-like appearance, or even absence of the ligament. Also, differentiation between the long head and the superior ligament may be difficult. The long head is sometimes membranous and at the attachment a synovial fold with villi may be observed. Villi can be seen mainly in the superior and inferior cavities.

At the bottom of the subacromial bursa, the upper surface of the rotator cuff can be observed.

CLINICAL EXPERIENCES

Arthroscopy of the shoulder joint had first been performed by Dr. Michael Burman (1931) and Prof. Kenji Takagi (1935). However, they were unable to apply arthroscopy to routine clinical cases. With the development by Prof. Masaki Watanabe of the No. 24 arthroscope in 1970, arthroscopy became suitable for routine clinical work.

From 1974 to 1982, 72 shoulder joints in 66 patients (44 male, 22 female) were examined by arthroscopy (Table 8). In addition, eight bursas (one subdeltoid bursa with

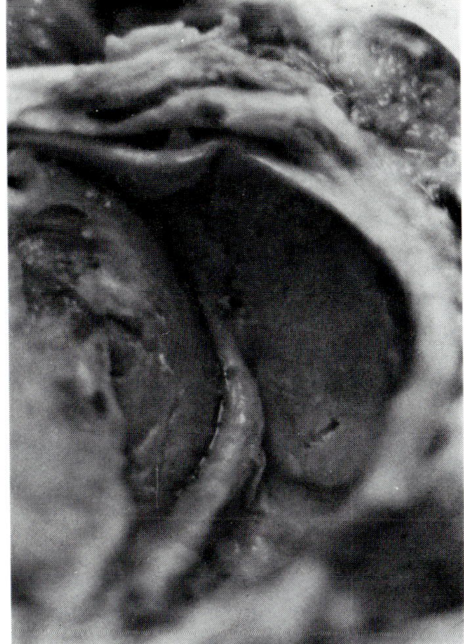

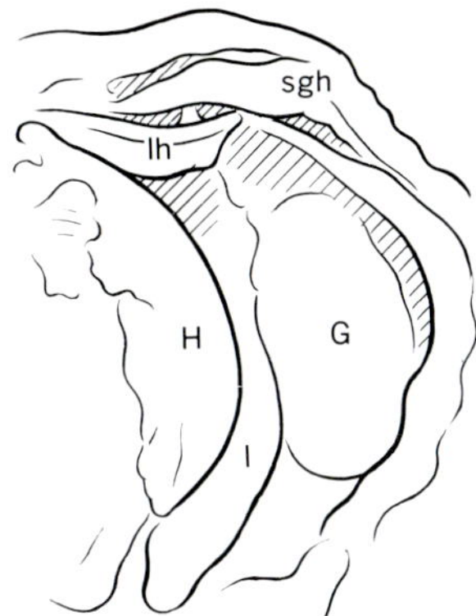

Fig. 54 Shoulder joint. (H) Humeral head. (G) Glenoid fossa. (lh) Long head of the brachial biceps. (l) Limbus. (sgh) Superior glenohumeral ligament.

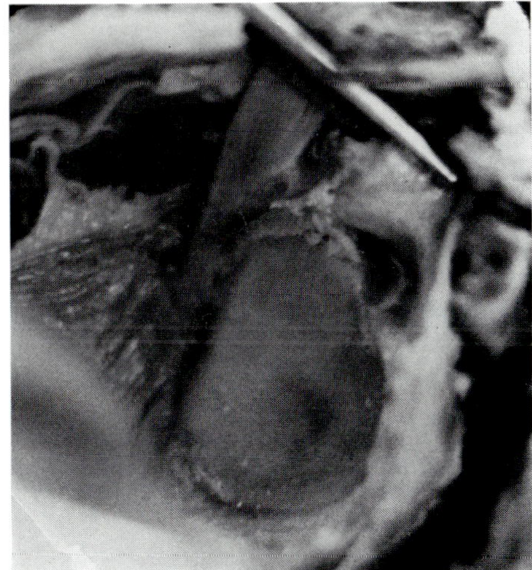

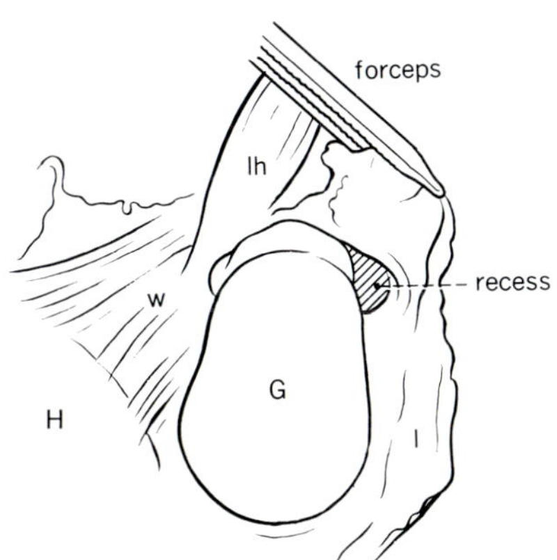

Fig. 55 Anterior recess. (G) Glenoid fossa. (H) Humeral head. (lh) Long head of the brachial biceps. (l) Limbus. (W) Posterior wall.

bursitis calcarea and seven subacromial bursas with rotator cuff injuries) and two acromioclavicular joints with dislocation were also examined with the No. 24 arthroscope (Table 9).

The oldest patient studied was a 69-year-old male and the youngest a 15-year-old female. The mean age was 40.8 years (male 39.0, female 49.8).

Of 84 arthroscopic examinations of shoulder joint, local anesthesia was used in 66, epidural anesthesia in 4, brachial plexus block in 11, and general anesthesia in 3.

Table 8 Arthroscopy of the shoulder joint

Diagnosis	Patients	Joints	Times
Pain	7	7	7
Sprain	5	5	5
Contracture	2	2	2
Snapping shoulder	6	6	6
Baseball shoulder	3	3	3
Rotator cuff injury	4	4	4
Biceps tendon rupture	3	3	4
Loose body	1	1	3
Loose shoulder	2	2	3
Recurrent dislocation	7	7	9
Frozen shoulder	6	6	6
Nonspecific arthritis	1	1	1
Rheumatoid arthritis	16	22	28
Reticulohistiocytosis	1	1	1
Bone cyst	1	1	1
Paralytic shoulder	1	1	1
Total	66	72	84

Table 9 Arthroscopic cases other than the shoulder joint

	Patients	Joints & bursas	Times
Subacromial bursa	7	7	7
Subdeltoid bursa	1	1	1
Acromioclavicular joint	2	2	2
Total	10	10	10

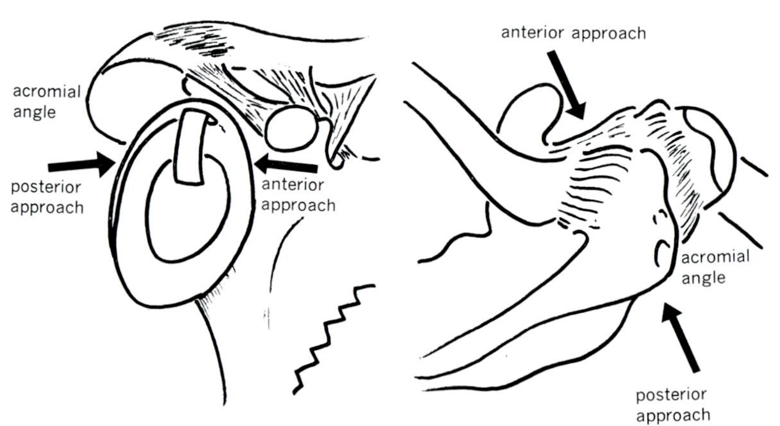

Fig. 56 Approaches.

Approaches to the shoulder joint used were the anterior, posterior, and combined. The anterior approach was used for 37 joints, the posterior for 34, and the combined for 13 (Fig. 56).

PROCEDURE

With posterior approach, insertion is about 1.5 to 2.0 cm below the acromial angle, and the angle of direction is with the tip of the coracoid process pointed horizontally. The tip of the needle reaches just below the junction of the biceps tendon and the glenoid process at the top of the glenohumeral joint through the deltoid muscle and the infraspinatus muscle. For the posterior approach, the lateral position can be used. Attention must be paid to the suprascapular artery, its acromial branch, and the suprascapular nerve, which are away from the route. Also, the axillary artery and the posterosuperior humeral circumflex artery have certain distance from the route.

The anterior approach is usually performed with the patient in the supine or sitting position. Raising the shoulder joint with a hard pillow under the back in the supine position and 45° abducted position facilitate the insertion. Insertion is in the lateral border of the coracoid process. The angle of direction is a right angle to the horizontal plane. In the case of an object located in the bottom of the joint cavity, insertion should be lower. The needle passes through the deltoid muscle and along the lateral border of the short head of the brachial biceps tendon. The branch of the axillary artery, the acromial branch of the thoracoacromial artery, the plexus of the acromial artery, and the deltoid muscle branch of the superior brachial circumflex artery are away from the route. Anterior, posterior, and even lateral approaches to the subacromial bursa can be applied with the patient in a sitting position. When using a supine position for anterior approach, it is sometimes necessary to put the arm in traction so that the anterior capsule pushes down on the anterior surface of the humeral head. If the anterior capsule is broken, it is difficult to make a diagnosis. Based on these observations, the sitting position is most convenient; however, occasionally the patient will complain of pain in the buttocks and the patient's clothes may be contaminated by the operator's hair. Therefore, it is best to use footholders so the patient can change the position of the buttocks, and to take care not to let the operator's cap touch the patient's clothes. With the sitting position, the visual field is wide and manipulation is easy.

The visual field of both approaches is shown in Figure 57. In the posterior approach,

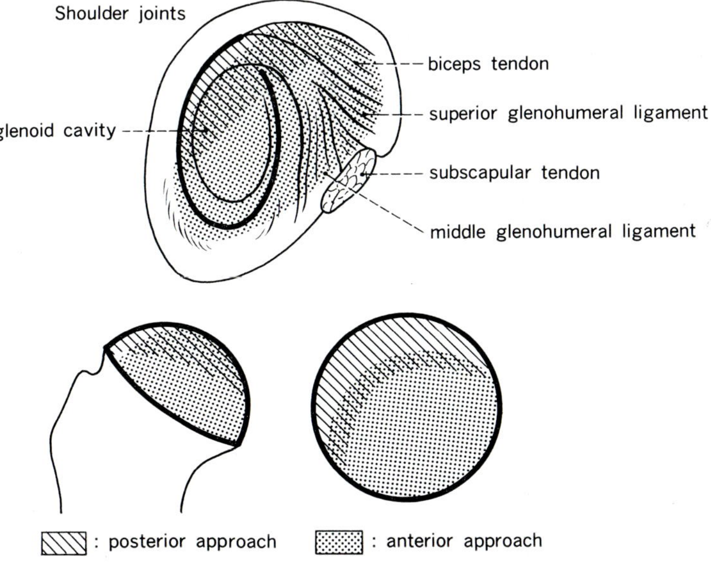

Fig. 57 Visible field in shoulder arthroscopy.

the distal portion of the long head of the brachial biceps tendon cannot be followed, as compared with the anterior approach.

CLINICAL CASES

Case 1 A 35-year-old man with pain on motion in the right shoulder joint (Fig. 58).
In October 1973, pain on motion occurred in the right shoulder joint without any difinite cause. In the first physical examination on May 27, 1974, anterior and lateral elevation more than 140 was painful without tenderness. On July 22, 1974, the arthroscopic examination through the anterior approach under local anesthesia revealed the thick and frayed rim of the limbus of the glenoid surface with irregularity of the surface of the humeral head.

Case 2 A 24-year-old man with pain on motion in the right shoulder joint (Fig. 59).
Three or four months before presentation, the patient had complained of pain at the moment of serving in tennis. The first physical examination on November 7, 1977, revealed click on motion without pain or without limitation of motion. The arthro-

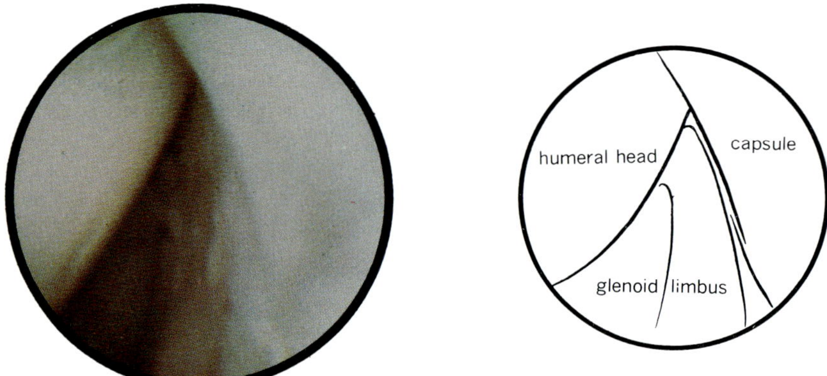

Fig. 58 Case 1. The thick and frayed inner rim of the limbus in the right shoulder joint, anterior approach.

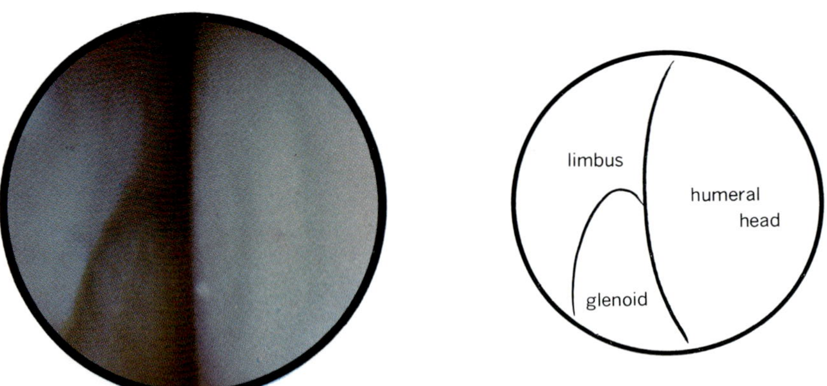

Fig. 59 Case 2. Degenerated limbus, posterior approach.

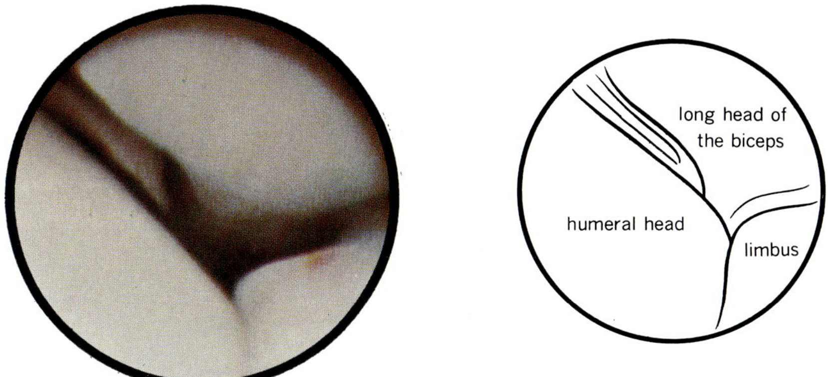

Fig. 60 Case 3. Anterior dislocation of the long head with a rupture of the superior glenohumeral ligament, anterior approach.

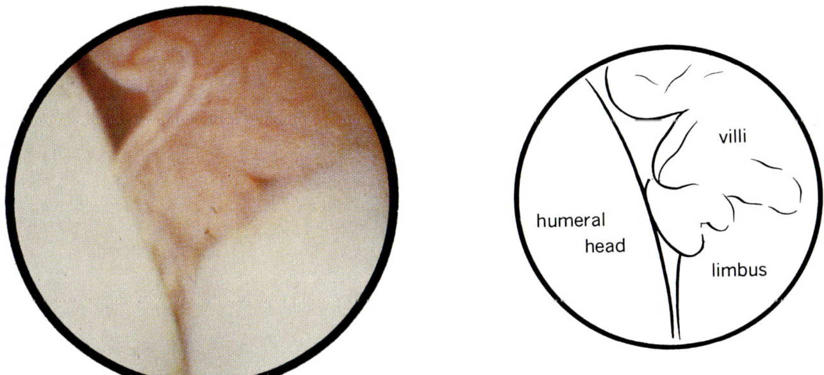

Fig. 61 Case 3. Villi proliferation (baseball shoulder), anterior approach.

scopic examination on November 18, 1977, revealed degenerated limbus with villi proliferation.

Case 3 A 32-year-old man with right baseball shoulder (Figs. 60 and 61).

For ten years before the first examination, the patient had complained of pain on motion in the right shoulder joint while playing baseball. In the first physical examination of June 20, 1979, the patient complained of pain at the maximum elevation without limitation of motion. On June 27, 1979, arthroscopic examination was performed through the anterior approach under local anesthesia. During the examination the ruptured end of the superior glenohumeral ligament along the long head and the anteriorly dislocated long head of the brachial biceps tendon were observed. The tip of the arthroscope easily reached the posterior upper wall of the joint through the rupture. There was villi proliferation in the superior cavity.

Case 4 A 29-year-old man with right baseball shoulder (Figs. 62–64).

The patient began playing baseball one year before presentation. Gradually, pain began to occur in the right shoulder. On a full power throw, pain was always felt in the shoulder. In the first physical examination on July 8, 1982, there was tenderness

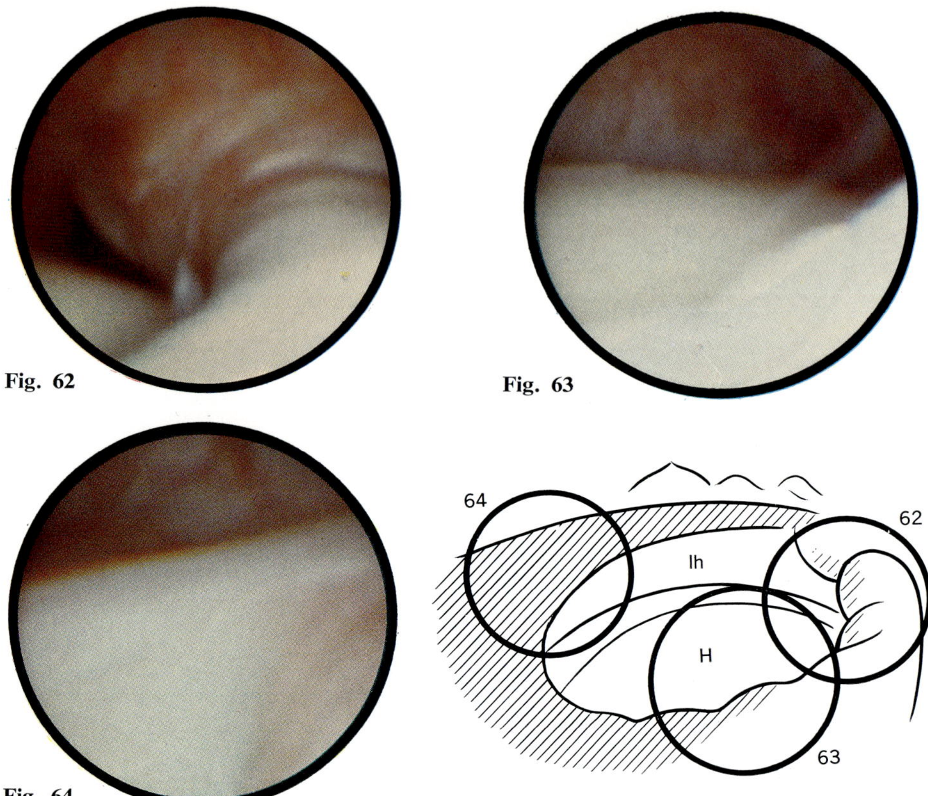

Fig. 62

Fig. 63

Fig. 64

Figs. 62, 63, 64 Case 4. Rupture of the anterior capsule (baseball shoulder), anterior approach. (lh) Long head of the brachial biceps. (H) Humeral head.

anteriorly and pain occurred on posterior raising with external rotation. On July 28, 1982, arthroscopic examination was performed through the anterior approach under local anesthesia in a sitting position. A thick cord-like tissue was observed in the front of the long head of the brachial biceps tendon. The distal portion of the tissue turned over laterally, ran back to the proximal portion, and eventually joined to the starting place. The anterior portion of the capsule had been broken. There was a wide space in the medial superior portion of the attached place of the long head of the biceps tendon due to rupture of the superior capsule.

Case 5 A 28-year-old man with right baseball shoulder (Figs. 65–67).

The patient experienced pain on a full power throw while playing baseball. In the first physical examination of July 13, 1982, pain occurred when the right arm was raised at 90° laterally with external rotation. There was tenderness at the posterior and anterior portion of the acromion. On August 11, 1982, arthroscopic examination was performed through the anterior approach in a sitting position. It was possible to follow the inner rim of the broken anterior capsule, which appeared as cord-like tissue. The opening of the subscapular bursa was observed at the anteroinferior portion of the glenoid process. In the bursa, a thick cord-like tissue surrounded with villi was observed. In the superior wall of the attachment of the long head of the biceps tendon, a rupture was observed. The tip of the arthroscope entered the chamber and villi and cord-like tissue were observed.

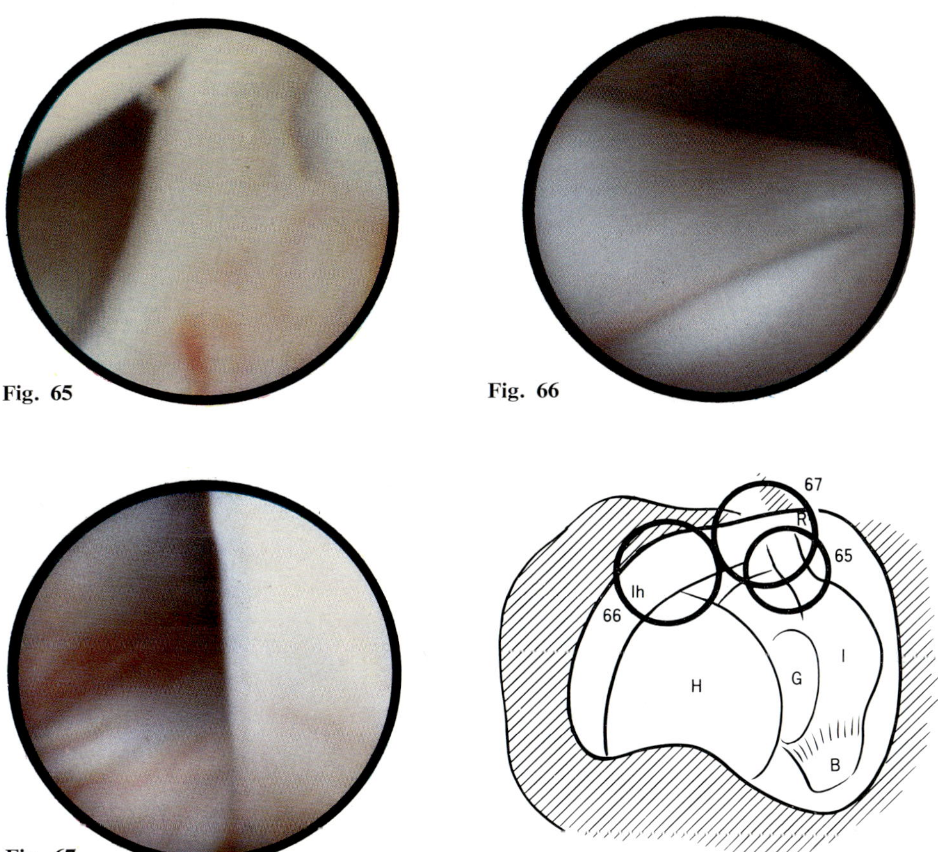

Figs. 65, 66, 67 Case 5. Baseball shoulder, anterior approach. (R) Upper medial cavity through the superior surface of the long head. (B) Subscapular bursa. (H) Humeral head. (G) Glenoid fossa. (lh) Long head of the brachial biceps. (l) Limbus.

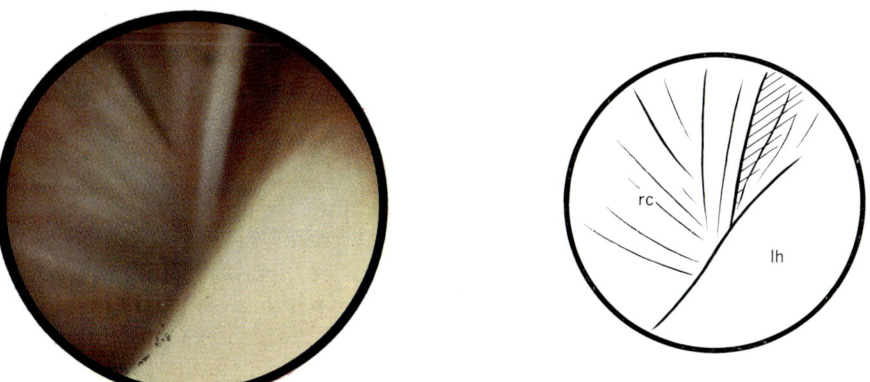

Fig. 68 Case 6. Recurrent dislocation of the right shoulder, anterior approach. (lh) Long head. (rc) Rotator cuff.

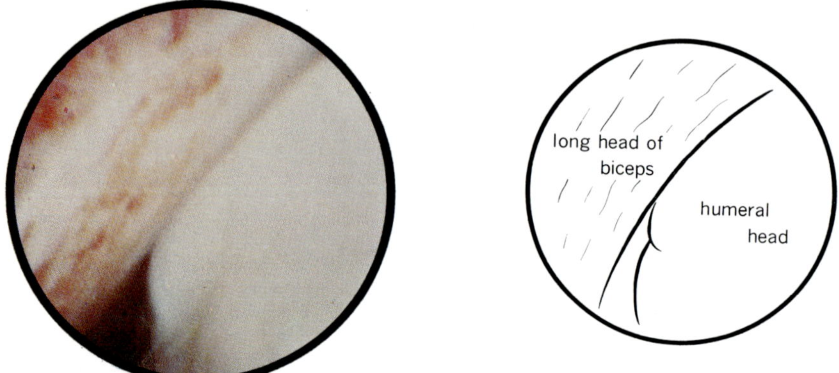

Fig. 69 Case 7. A bulge of the articular surface of the humeral head with the hyperemic long head of the biceps, anterior approach.

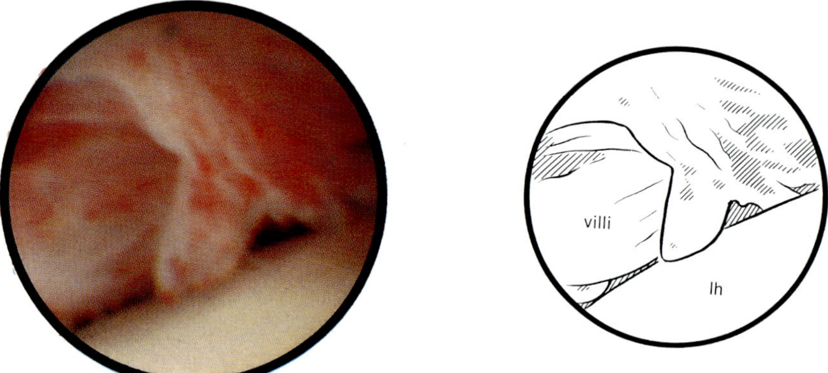

Fig. 70 Case 8. Rheumatoid arthritis, anterior approach. (lh) Long head.

The other three cases of baseball shoulder that were operated upon revealed the same findings in arthroscopy as the above cases. The anterior capsule with a part of the subscapular muscle tendon was ruptured. It was sutured in the surgery.

Case 6 A 20-year-old man with recurrent dislocation of the right shoulder joint (Fig. 68). One year before presentation, the right shoulder joint was dislocated while doing Japanese sumo wrestling. Since then, the joint has been dislocated several times. In the first physical examination on May 28, 1981, anterior raising was restricted at 65°. On July 31, 1981, arthroscopic examination was performed through the anterior approach under local anesthesia. The anteroinferior portion of the limbus was defective. It was possible to introduce the tip of the arthroscope into the medial direction through the upper part of the attachment of the long head because the superior capsule was broken. A part of the rotator cuff could be seen through the synovium. During arthroscopy, the long head was snapped.

Case 7 A 54-year-old man with periarthritis of the left shoulder (Fig. 69). In May 1977, the patient had pain in the left shoulder. On January 17, 1978, the first physical examination revealed slight limitation of external rotation and anterior elevation with tenderness in the anterior area. On July 21, 1978, arthroscopic examina-

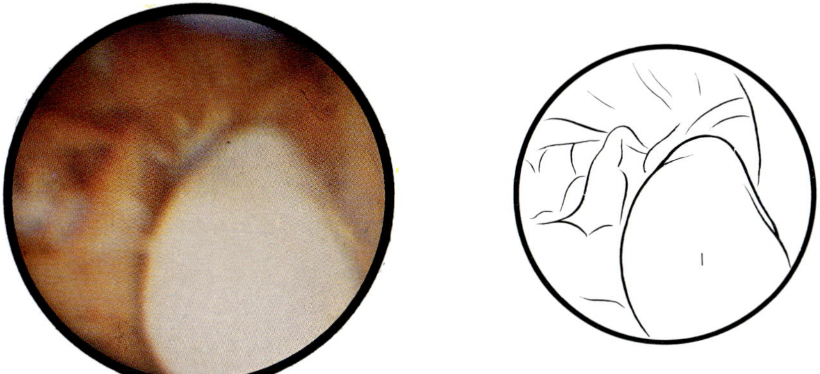

Fig. 71 Case 9. A loose body, anterior approach. (I) A loose body.

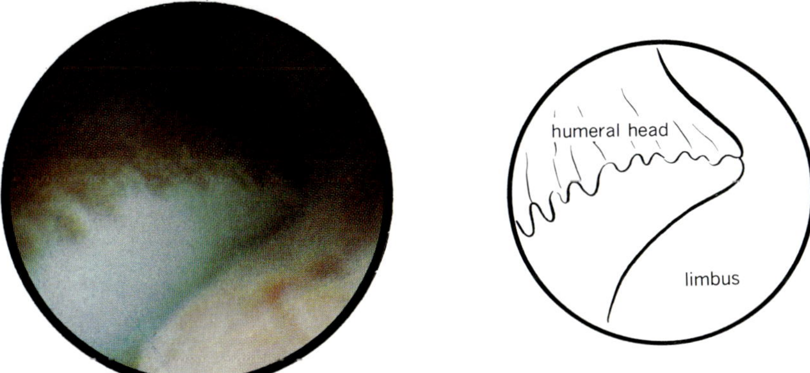

Fig. 72 Case 10. Pannus formation of the humeral head, posterior approach (Picture taken by Dr. M. Watanabe.).

tion through an anterior approach under local anesthesia revealed a bulge of the articular surface of the humeral head with the hyperemic long head of the biceps tendon.

Case 8 A 69-year-old woman with rheumatoid arthritis in the left shoulder joint (Fig. 70). Arthroscopic examination was performed on October 26, 1981. The anterior approach was applied. A proliferation of hyperemic villi was observed.

Case 9 A 17-year-old boy with a loose body in the right shoulder joint (Fig. 71). Ten days before the first examination, while practicing judo, the patient's partner fell on the right shoulder of the patient. For three days the patient could not raise his right arm more than 120°. In the first physical examination on August 15, 1980, there were no specific findings. On November 2, 1980, the same shoulder was twisted postero-superiorly. On November 5, 1980, the diagnosis was made. On September 3, 1981, a loose body was removed by Dr. Kazuaki Yajima under arthroscopic control with the patient in a sitting position.

Case 10 A 42-year-old man with bone cyst of the glenoid process on the left (Fig. 72). One year before presentation, dull pain occurred in the patient's left shoulder without any apparent cause. On July 7, 1975, in the first physical examination, the above diagnosis was made. On September 12, 1975, arthroscopic examination of the left shoulder joint through the posterior approach under local anesthesia revealed a pannus formation in the humeral head.

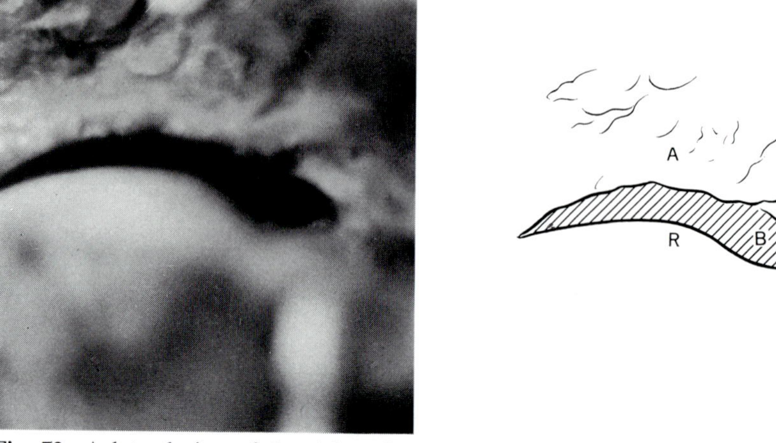

Fig. 73 A lateral view of the right subacromial bursa. The acromion was resected. (A) Acromion. (B) Subacromial bursa. (R) Rotator cuff.

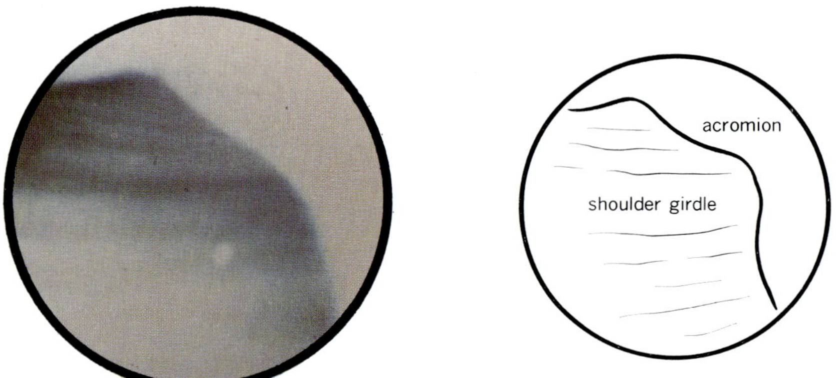

Fig. 74 Case 11. Shoulder girdle in the subacromial bursa, lateral approach.

SUBACROMIAL BURSAS

The subacromial bursa is between the acromion at the top and the rotator cuff at the bottom (Fig. 73). The trocar is inserted laterally.

Case 11 A 24-year-old woman with strain in the acromioclavicular joint on the left (Fig. 74).

On July 21, 1978, after the patient fell down, pain occurred in the left shoulder. On the same day, in the first physical examination, the patient complained of pain while bringing down the left arm laterally after anterior elevation. On July 27, 1978, arthroscopic examination of the subacromial bursa under local anesthesia was performed through the lateral approach. The rotator cuff was well observed.

Case 12 A 14-year-old boy with right baseball shoulder (Fig. 75).

One week before presentation, the patient experienced pain when he threw a ball. In the first physical examination on June 14, 1982, anterior and lateral raising

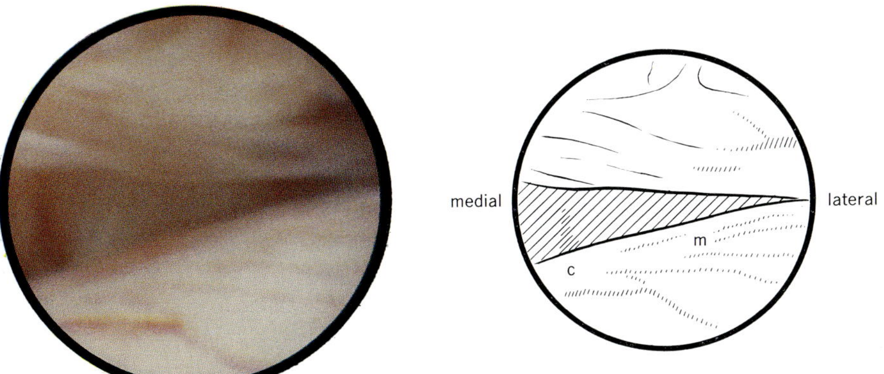

Fig. 75 Case 12. The right subacromial bursa. A cord-like tissue in the medial side becomes membranous in the lateral side. Posterolateral approach. (c) Cord-like tissue. (m) Membranous tissue.

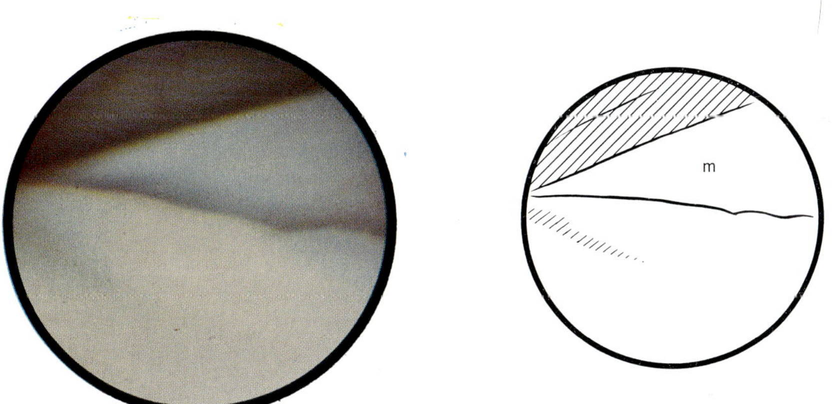

Fig. 76 Case 13. (Same patient as in Figs. 65–67): Baseball shoulder, lateral approach. (m) Membranous tissue.

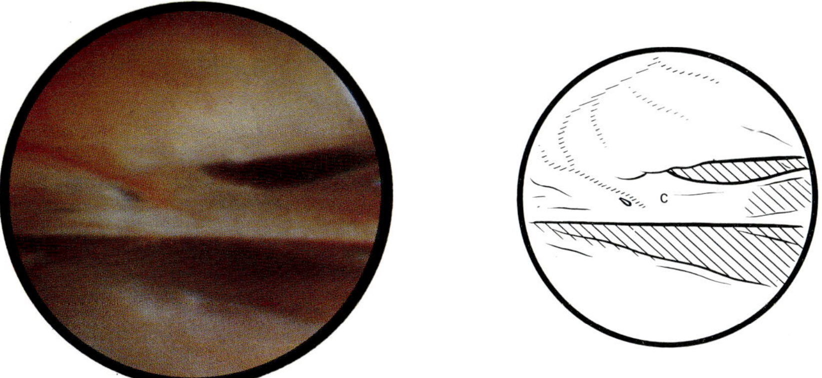

Fig. 77 Case 14. (Same patient as in Fig. 70): Rheumatoid arthritis, lateral approach. (c) Cord-like tissue.

was restricted. On July 14, 1982, arthroscopic examination of the right glenohumeral joint and subacromial bursa was performed. In the joint, dislocation of the long head of the brachial biceps tendon was observed. In the bursa, a cord-like tissue running to the lateral transversely was observed; however, it was impossible to discern its clinical significance.

Case 13 A 28-year-old man (Fig. 76).

This is the same patient as in Case 5, shoulder joint. Lateral approach was applied. Anteriorly membranous tissue was observed.

Case 14 A 69-year-old woman (Fig. 77).

This is the same patient as in Case 8, shoulder joint. The lateral approach was applied. A cord-like tissue with hyperemia was observed.

5

Arthroscopy of the Elbow Joint

In a large number of patients with complaints involving the elbow joint, diagnosis has been difficult, as it is for other joint diseases. Diagnosis of lesions of the elbow joint should be based on both history and clinical findings, especially. X-rays in several directions, with arthrography, are useful for diagnosis. But intraarticular lesions of the joint should be diagnosed through direct methods of investigation.

In 1970, Watanabe developed the No. 24 arthroscope, and now arthroscopy of the small joints has been developed for clinical use. But there are few reports of arthroscopy of the elbow joint because of its anatomic complexity. In 1931, Dr. Burman reported arthroscopy of the small joints of cadavers using his endoscope (3.0 mm in diameter). He stated that "the elbow joint is another of the large joints unsuitable for examination, since the joint space is so narrow for the relatively large needle. The anterior puncture of the elbow is out of the question and the midposterior puncture is poor for our purpose."

In 1971, Watanabe reported the clinical use of the 1.7–mm diameter No. 24 arthroscope for small joints. The author (1979, 1980a) reported that the transligamentous posteroradial approach (posterior radial approach) is suitable for routine elbow joint arthroscopy because it offers the widest visible fields. The author (1980b) also reported the arthroscopic anatomy of the elbow joint and six approaches used in a cadaver study. At the same time, Maeda (1980) reported on the transtendinous posterior approach for the purpose of inspection of the posterior part of the joint cavity. In 1981 the author reported the clinical study of the elbow joint arthroscopy based on 226 cases. Today, arthroscopic examination of the elbow joint has been developed to the stage of clinical use.

ARTHROSCOPIC ANATOMY OF THE ELBOW JOINT

The anatomy of the elbow joint as seen through the arthroscope is not at all comparable to that seen by dissection. The conventional concepts presented in anatomy textbooks cannot be directly utilized during arthroscopy (Fig. 78). Under normal circumstances, the elbow joint contains neither large quantities of fluid nor gas, and also vacuous spaces do not exist. By filling the joint with normal saline or gas, the situation is altered considerably. For understanding and recording the arthroscopic findings, detailed anatomy of the joint cavity is essential (Fig. 79). Figure 80 shows the detailed arthroscopic anatomy of the elbow joint.

The elbow joint is an intermediate joint of the upper limb, which is composed of the distal end of the humerus, the olecranon of the ulna, and the radius head. As shown in Table 10, the elbow joint can be subdivided arthroscopically into four interspaces (the humeroulnar, humeroradial, proximal radioulnar, and radioannular interspaces); and six synovial pouches (the medial synovial and lateral synovial pouches, the sacciform recess, and the radial, coronoid, and olecranon fossae).

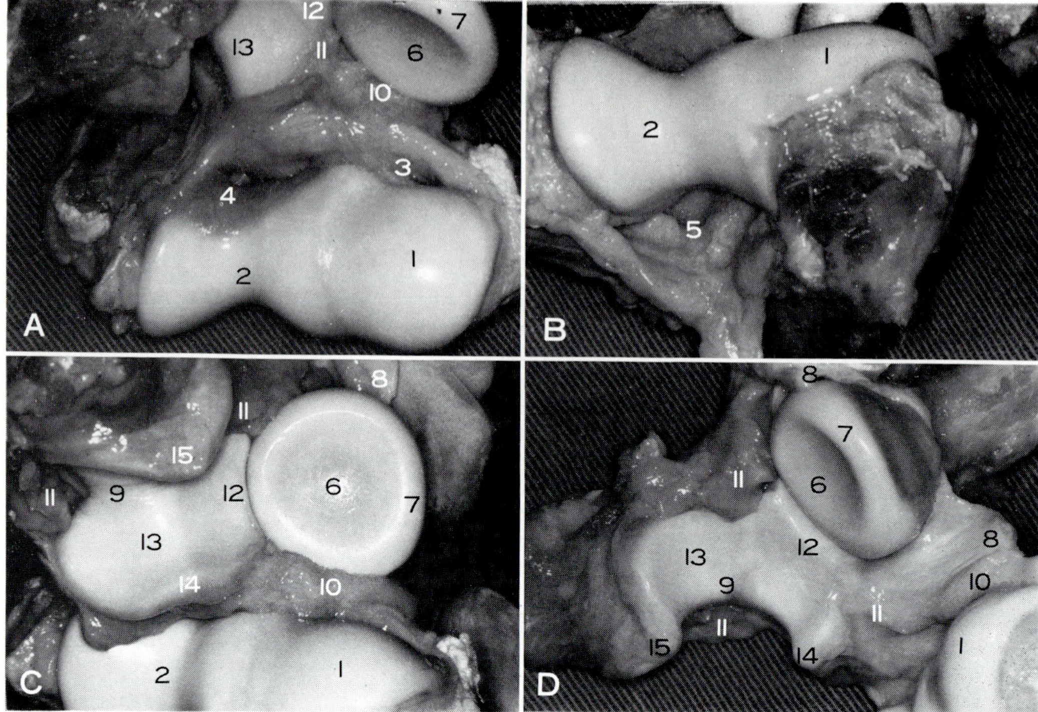

Fig. 78 Cross section through the elbow joint.
(A) Anterior view of humeral condyle.
(B) Posterior view of humeral condyle.
(C) Head of radius and ulna.
(D) Side view.

1. Capitulum
2. Trochlea
3. Radial fossa
4. Coronoid fossa
5. Olecranon fossa
6. Head of radius
7. Articular circumference
8. Annular ligament
9. Nonarticular area
10. Synovial fold
11. Synovial fat pad
12. Radial notch of ulna
13. Trochlear notch of ulna
14. Coronoid process
15. Olecranon

Fig. 79 Detailed anatomy of the elbow joint.

1. Depression of the radius head
2. Marginal zone of the radius head
3. Articular circumference
4. Circumferential synovial fold
5. Annular ligament
6. Tongue-like synovial fat pad
7. Proximal radioulnar interspace
8. Radial notch of the ulna
9. Transverse sulcus of the trochlear notch (nonarticular area)
10. Capitulum
11. Trochlea
12. Intercondylar eminence
13. Radial fossa
14. Coronoid fossa
15. Olecranon fossa
16. Sacciform recess
17. Synovial fat pad
18. Transverse fibrous cord
19. Coronoid process
20. Olecranon
21. Trochlear notch of the ulna
22. Central eminence of the trochlear notch
23. Triangular synovial fold

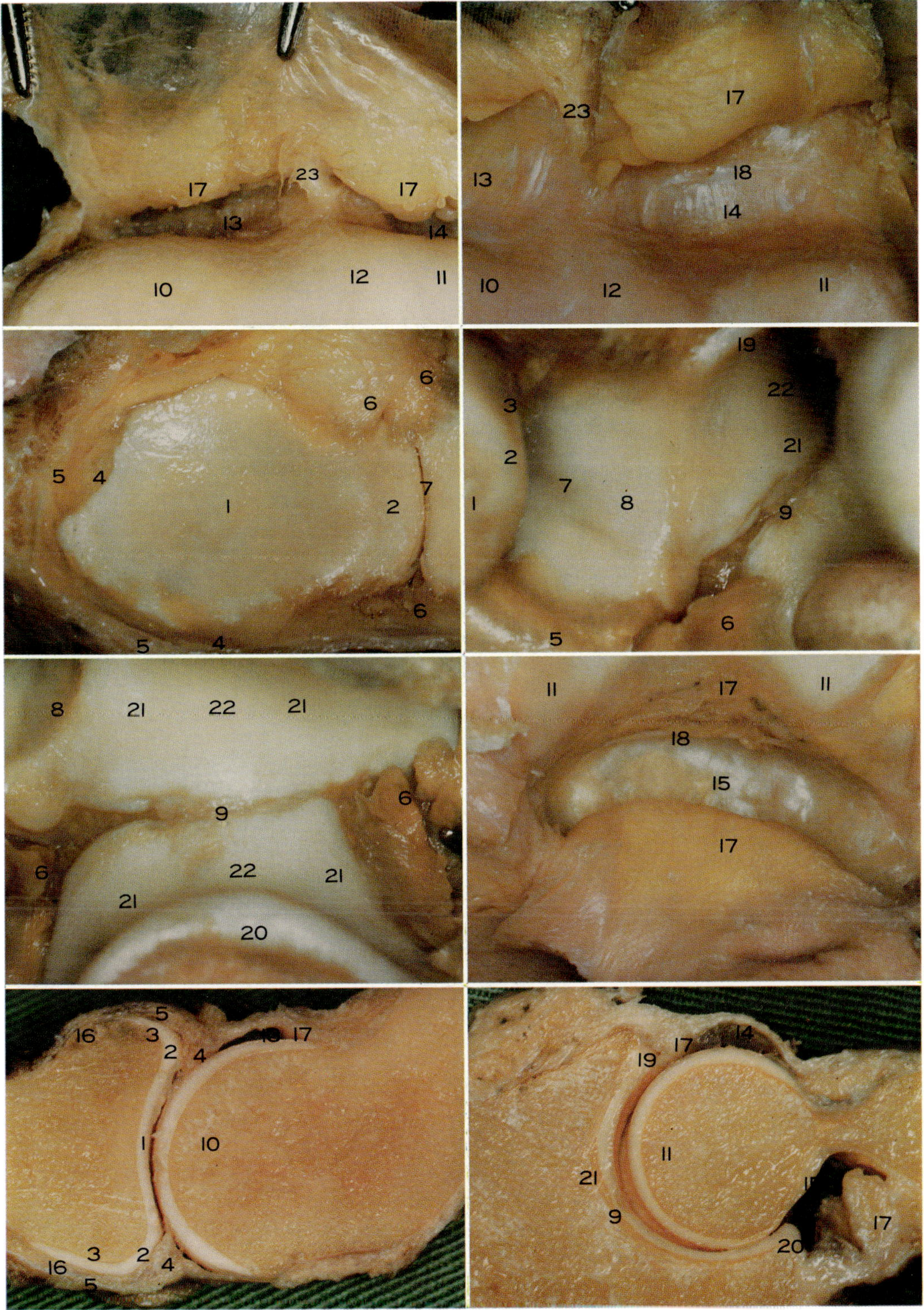

Fig. 79 (Legends on opposite page.)

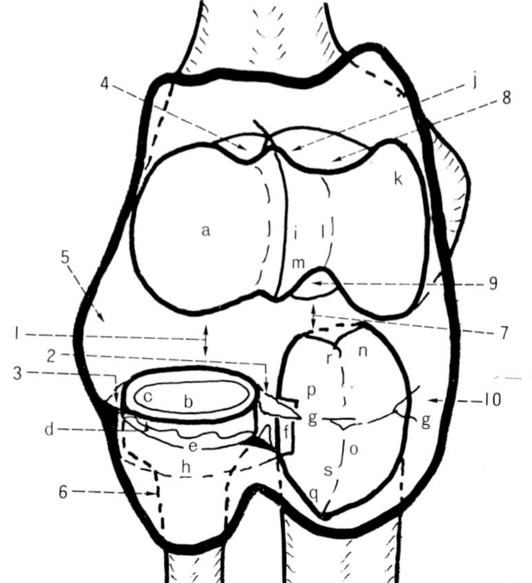

1. Humeroradial interspace.
2. Aproximal radioulnar interspace.
3. Radioannular interspace.
4. Radial fossa.
5. Lateral synovial pouch.
6. Sacciform recess.
7. Humeroulnar interspace.
8. Coronoid fossa.
9. Olecranon fossa.
10. Medial synovial pouch.

a. Humeral capitulum.
b. Depression of the head of radius.
c. Marginal zone of the head of radius.
d. Circumferential synovial fold.
e. Articular circumference.
f. Radial notch of the ulna.
g. Tongue-like fat pad.
h. Annular ligament.
i. Intercondylar eminence.
j. Triangular synovial fold.
k. Medial convex articular facet of the trochlea.
l. Trochlear sulcus.
m. Lateral convex articular facet of the trochlea.
n. Medial concave articular facet of the trochlear notch.
o. Transverse sulcus of the trochlear notch.
p. Lateral concave articular facet of the trochlear notch.
q. Coronoid process.
r. Olecranon.
s. Central eminence of the trochlear notch.

Fig. 80 Arthroscopic anatomy of the elbow joint.

The capsule is attached proximally to the upper margins of the radial fossa, the coronoid fossa, the olecranon fossa, and the humeral capitulum, and distally to the anterior, posterior, and medial margins of the ulnar trochlear notch. It is also attached laterally to the neck of the radius head and the distal margin of the ulnar radial notch, wrapping the radius head. The medial collateral ligament strengthens the medial side of the joint and the lateral collateral ligament strengthens the lateral side. The quadrate ligament is square-shaped, reinforcing the sacciform recess from below. It is stretched distally between the radial notch of the ulna and the articular circumference of the radius head. The annular ligament is a strong fibrocartilaginous ring-shaped band that surrounds the articular circumference of the radius head, and the inside of this ligament is covered with cartilage. The inner side of the capsular ligament, except for the inside of the annular ligament, is covered with the synovial membrane.

There are two articular surfaces at the distal end of the humerus; i.e., the humeral trochlea on the ulnar side, and the humeral capitulum on the radial side. The humeral trochlea is spool-shaped, and the articular cartilage expands from the anterior to the posterior, covering the distal end. The depression called the trochlear groove runs longitudinally through its center. Both sides of the trochlear groove are elevated and gently curved, and are known as the convex facets of the trochlea. The humeral capitulum is ball-shaped,

Table 10 Subdivision of the elbow joint

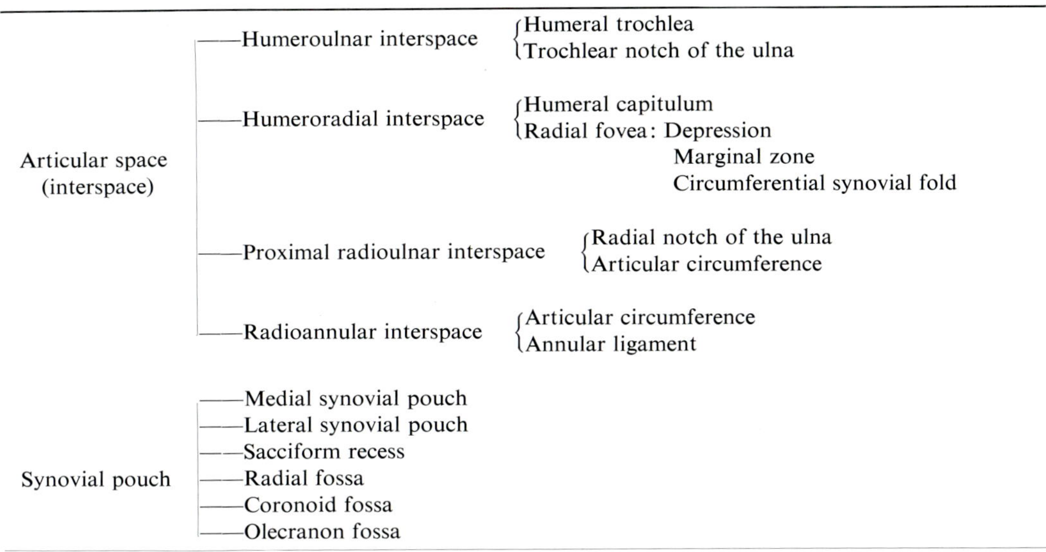

Part	Subdivision	Components
Articular space (interspace)	Humeroulnar interspace	Humeral trochlea; Trochlear notch of the ulna
	Humeroradial interspace	Humeral capitulum; Radial fovea: Depression, Marginal zone, Circumferential synovial fold
	Proximal radioulnar interspace	Radial notch of the ulna; Articular circumference
	Radioannular interspace	Articular circumference; Annular ligament
Synovial pouch	Medial synovial pouch	
	Lateral synovial pouch	
	Sacciform recess	
	Radial fossa	
	Coronoid fossa	
	Olecranon fossa	

with articular cartilage from the anterior to the posterior half of the distal end of the humerus. The humeral trochlea articulates with the ulnar trochlear notch, whereas the humeral capitulum articulates with the fovea of the radius head.

The trochlear notch of the ulna is warped and roof-shaped in an anteroposterior direction, and semicircular from side to side. In its center, the peak-shaped elevation runs longitudinally from the olecranon to the coronoid process, which is known as the central eminence of the trochlear notch and corresponds to the trochlear groove. Both dented slopes of this ridge, called the concave facets of the trochlear notch, articulate with the convex facets of the trochlea. The olecranon is inserted into the olecranon fossa, situated at the posterior side of the humerus during extension of the elbow joint. The coronoid process inserts into the coronoid fossa, situated at the anterior side of the humerus during flexion. The radial notch articulates with the articular circumference of the radius head, which lies just lateral to the distal margin of the trochlear notch in an anteroposterior direction. Almost in the middle of the trochlear notch, the drain-shaped nonarticulating area, known as the transverse sulcus in the trochlear notch, runs transversely in various forms and sizes. The synovial membrane and two tongue-like adiposynovial flinges overlie this sulcus. No cartilage is present in the adult elbow joint.

The radial fovea, the depression of the radius head, is cup-shaped with a shallow sunken center. The peripheral margin of this depression, the marginal zone of the radius head, looks like a narrow convex slope, on which the ring-shaped circumferential synovial folds, in various forms and sizes, are overlaid. They articulate with the humeral capitulum, and some of them insert into the radial fossa situated at the anterior part of the humerus when the elbow joint flexes. The articular circumference consists of the proximal radioulnar joint with the ulnar radial notch, and also the joint-like articulation with the annular ligament.

The lateral pouch is situated at the lateral side of the humeroradial joint, and the medial pouch is situated at the medial side of the humeroulnar joint. There is a large amount of synovial villi in these two pouches and the sacciform recess. Also, synovial fat pads with villi are found in the three fossae, i.e., the olecranon fossa, coronoid fossa, and radial fossa. The tongue-like adiposynovial flinges are seen on the proximal radioulnar joint space and on both sides of the transverse sulcus in the trochlear notch.

APPROACHES AND VISIBLE FIELDS

There are several approaches for insertion of the arthroscope. Six approaches are suitable for arthroscopy of the elbow joint (Fig. 81). These approaches and their visible fields are shown in Figures 82–87. The approach routinely used is the posterior radial approach because it gives the widest view and easy manipulation of the arthroscope in the joint cavity.

Anterior Radial Approach (Fig. 82)

This approach is suitable for examination of the anterior part of the joint. With the elbow joint flexed at a right angle, the depression between the humeral capitulum, the radius head, and the anterior margin of the lateral collateral ligament can be palpated with the examiner's thumb. The entry point is the center of this depression. The anterior half of the humeral capitulum, the fovea of the radius head, the lateral half of the humeroulnar, the radial fossa, the coronoid fossa, the anterior third of the medial pouch, and the lateral pouch are clearly visible.

Posterior Radial Approach (Fig. 83)

The most satisfactory site for the insertion of an arthroscope is the triangular gap on the posterior radial side of the joint. With the elbow joint flexed at a right angle, this easy-to-find triangular gap on the lateral side is the entry point for this approach. With the thumb, the examiner can palpate the depression that is circumscribed proximally by the lateral border of the humeral capitulum, distally by the edge of the radius head, and posteriorly

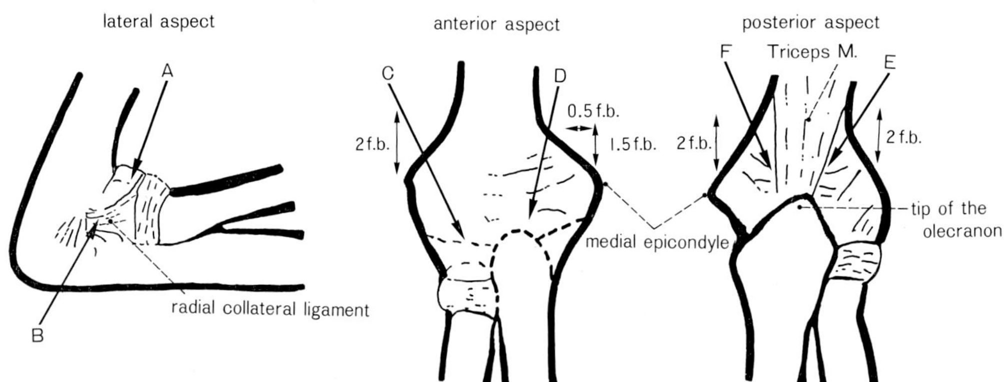

Fig. 81 Entry points and positions of the elbow joint.

A. Anterior radial approach. Elbow, 90° flexed. Forearm, neutral position.

B. Transligamentous posterior radial approach. Elbow, 90° flexed. Forearm, neutral position.

C. Anterolateral supracondylar approach. Elbow, 30° flexed. Forearm, external rotation.

D. Anteromedial supracondylar approach. Elbow, 45° flexed. Forearm, external rotation.

E. Posterolateral supraolecranal approach. Elbow, 60° flexed. Forearm, external rotation.

F. Posteromedial supraolecranal appraoch. Elbow, 90° flexed. Forearm, external rotation.

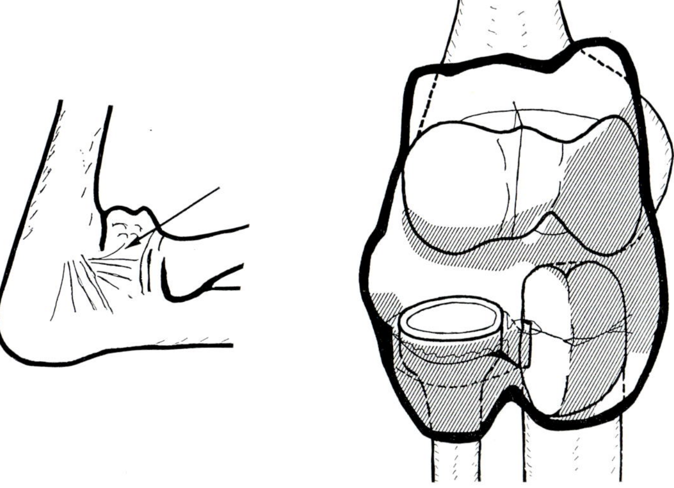

Fig. 82 Visible fields by anterior radial approach. Dark areas are difficult to observe.

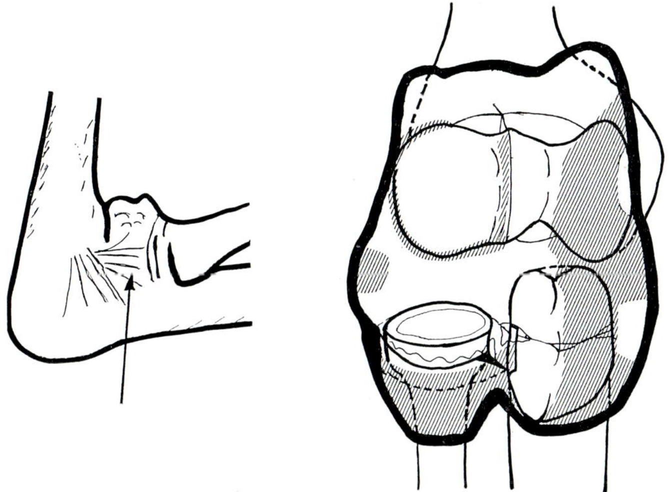

Fig. 83 Visible fields by posterior radial approach. Dark areas are difficult to observe.

by the lateral edge of the trochlear notch. This approach allows examination of almost the entire joint, except for the medial half of the humeroulnar joint and sacciform recess. The humeroradial joint and the lateral half of the humeroulnar interspace are clearly exposed. Satisfactory assessment of the proximal radioulnar joint and the articulation of the radial annular ligament is also possible via this approach. The radial fossa, the coronoid fossa, the olecranon fossa, and the middle third of the medial pouch can also be examined. But the tip of the coronoid process, the tip of the olecranon, the posterior half of the medial pouch, and a part of the lateral pouch cannot be fully inspected. Also, the medial half of the humeroulnar interspace and the sacciform recess cannot be observed by this approach.

Anterolateral Supracondylar Approach (Fig. 84)

This approach is suitable for examination of the anterolateral part of the joint. With the elbow joint flexed at 30°, the trocar puncture is made at two fingerbreadth proximal to

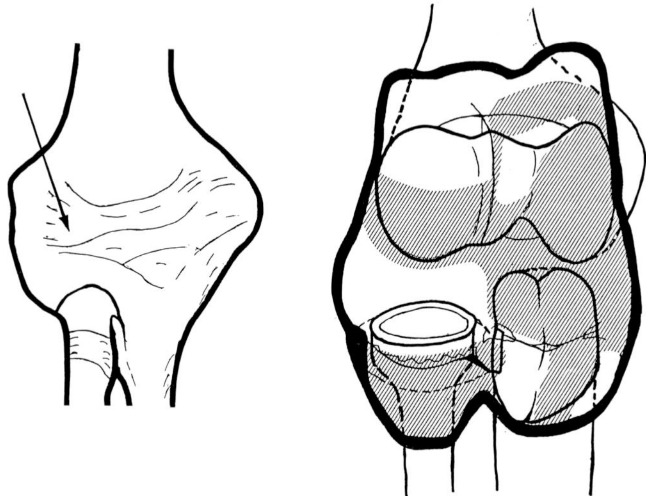

Fig. 84 Visible fields by anterolateral supracondylar approach. Dark areas are difficult to observe.

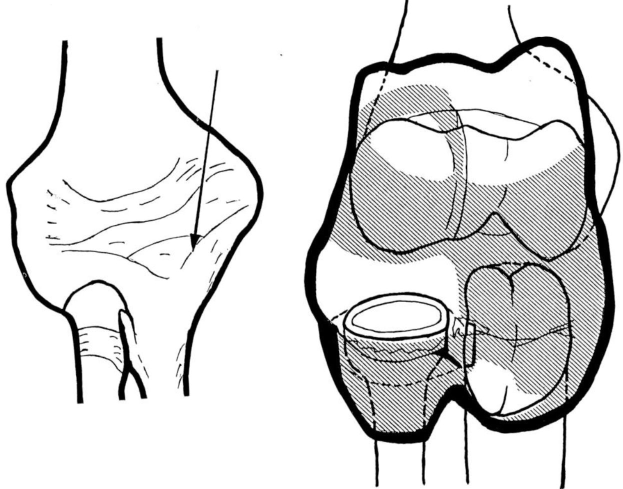

Fig. 85 Visible fields by anteromedial supracondylar approach. Dark areas are difficult to observe.

the lateral humeral epicondyle at its anterior aspect. The radial fossa, the lateral synovial pouch, the proximal radioulnar joint, the radial fovea, and the articulation of the radial annular ligament can be well examined.

Anteromedial Supracondylar Approach (Fig. 85)

This approach is especially suitable for the observation of the tip of the coronoid process, the anterior third of the humeroulnar interspace, the coronoid fossa, the lateral pouch, and the articulation of the proximal radioulnar joint. With the elbow joint flexed at 45°, the trocar puncture is made at the 1.5 fingerbreadth proximal to the medial humeral epicondyle.

Supraolecranal Approaches (Figs. 86 and 87)

These approaches are particularly suitable for observation of the tip of the olecranon, the posterior part of the humeroulnar interspace, and the olecranon fossa. With the elbow joint flexed at 60° for the posterolateral approach, and flexed 90° for the posteromedial approach, the trocar punctures are made at two fingerbreadth proximal to the superior end of the olecranon on both sides of the triceps muscle. Particular care must be taken to protect the ulnar nerve during the posteromedial supraolecranal approach.

There are certain "dead spaces," that is, spaces beyond the view of any approach, because of the complexity of the humeroulnar joint. For instance, two thirds of the medial humeroulnar joint and the sacciform recess are in the dead space of any approach. The amount of dead space will be reduced by improvements in arthroscopic technique through experience, and through the development of new approaches and better scopes.

The posterior radial approach is used in routine arthroscopy and another approach is combined for the purposes of detailed observation. These are shown in Table 11.

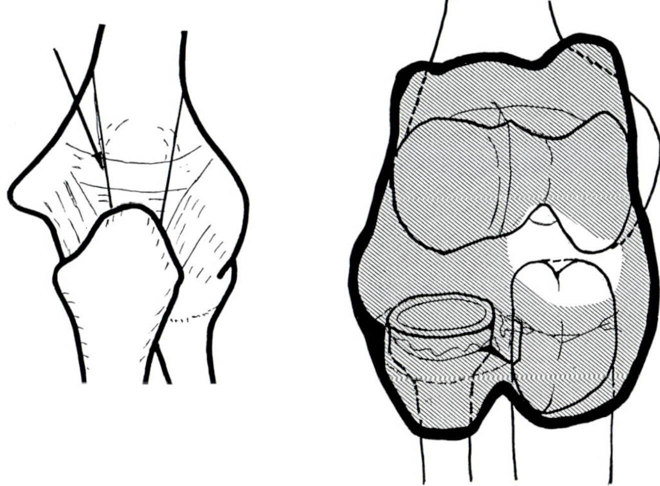

Fig. 86 Visible fields by posteromedial supraolecranal approach. Dark areas are difficult to observe.

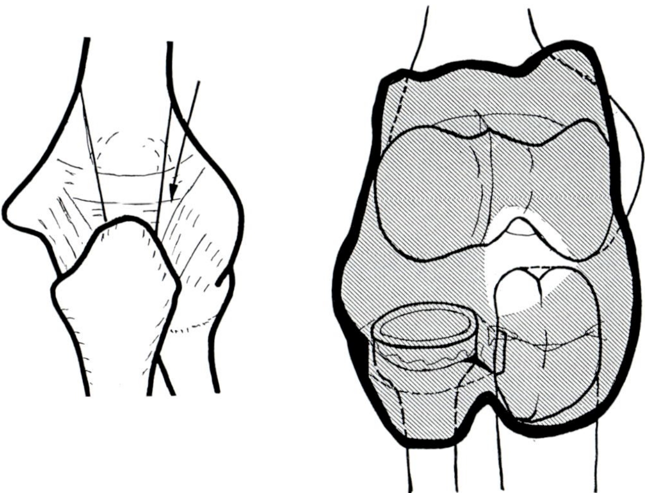

Fig. 87 Visible fields by posterolateral supraolecranal approach. Dark areas are difficult to observe.

Table 11 Approaches in elbow joint arthroscopy and visible field.

Anatomic detail examined	Approach					
	Anterior radial	Posterior radial	Anterolateral supracondylar	Anteromedial supracondylar	Posterolateral supraolecranal	Posteromedial supraolecranal
Humeral capitulum	++	++	+	+	–	–
Radial fovea	++	++	++	++	–	–
Circumferential synovial fold	++	++	++	++	–	–
Articular circumference	+	++	+	+	–	–
Radial notch of the ulna	+	+	+	+	–	–
Annular ligament	+	++	+	+	–	–
Medial convex facet of the trochlea	–	–	–	+	+	+
Trochlear groove	+	++	+	+	–	–
Lateral convex facet of the trochlea	+	++	+	+	+	+
Medial concave facet of the trochlear notch	–	–	–	+	–	+
Transverse sulcus of the trochlear notch	++	++	+	–	–	–
Lateral concave facet of the trochlear notch	++	++	+	+	+	+
Coronoid process	+	+	+	++	–	–
Olecranon	+	+	–	–	++	++
Central eminence of the trochlear notch	++	++	+	+	–	–
Radial fossa	++	++	++	+	–	–
Coronoid fossa	++	++	+	++	–	–
Olecranon fossa	+	++	+	+	++	++
Lateral synovial pouch	++	+	++	++	–	–
Medial synovial pouch	+	+	+	+	–	–
Sacciform recess	–	–	–	+	–	–

++ = Well observed. + = Difficult to observe. – = Impossible to observe.

BASIC TECHNIQUE

The fundamental techniques for arthroscopy of the elbow joint are very similar to those for other small joints, but the following important points should be noted. Because the elbow joint is an intricate and narrow-spaced joint, careful entry into the joint cavity and gentle manipulation of the arthroscope should be ensured.

Because a single puncture approach does not permit whole-area observation of the interior of the elbow joint, selection of an appropriate approach and the combination of several different approaches are necessary. Depending on the approach selected, it is very important that the joint be distended to the maximum with normal saline solution. An accurate puncture should be carried out carefully and gently with the aid of an obturator both at the time of the arthroscope's introduction into the joint and during change of position through elbow manipulation.

Having chosen the site for the insertion of the arthroscope, an 18-gauge lumbar puncture needle is inserted into the elbow joint. Any effusion should be aspirated. The joint capsule is fully distended for the trocar puncture by injection through this needle of 15 ml to 20 ml of normal saline at room temperature. The operator then makes a stab skin incision (2 mm to 3 mm) with a pointed scalpel. When the posterior radial approach is used, the elbow joint is flexed at 90° and the forearm pronated. The operator inserts the instrument in an anteromedial direction toward the humeroradial joint space. On no account should the sharp needle be allowed to deeply enter the joint cavity, as it may easily injure the articular cartilage. When the operator feels that the capsule has been penetrated, the sharp needle is exchanged for a blunt one. Then the sheath with the blunt needle is pushed into the joint cavity. Assuming that the sheath is precisely positioned in the joint cavity, the blunt needle can be exchanged for the arthroscope. The infusion fluid supply tube with the syringe, or the carbon dioxide inflation supply tube, is connected to the side hole of the sheath. Sufficient expantion of the joint space by the pressure of the normal saline or gas should be observed through the arthroscope. If the visual field is obstructed by the villi, etc., covering the front of the scope, these can be removed by stronger pressure. When moving the instrument to and fro, the arthroscope must be exchanged for the blunt needle.

CLINICAL ARTHROSCOPY

Anesthesia for Arthroscopy

The elbow joint can be anesthetized by infiltration with a 0.5% solution of a local anesthetic agent at the site of the insertion of the arthroscope. All tissue layers from the skin to the joint capsule must be fully anesthetized. A lumbar puncture needle, 18-gauge or larger, is inserted into the joint space and the elbow joint is filled with a 2% solution of local anesthetics. Approximately 15 ml to 20 ml local anesthetic is sufficient for intraarticular anesthesia of the elbow joint. The operator should wait about 5 minutes for the anesthesia to become fully effective for arthroscopy. The intraarticular anesthesia remains effective for at least 45 minutes. General, conduction, and intravenous anesthesia are of course usable, but intraarticular anesthesia has the following advantages for elbow joint arthroscopy:

1. The investigation can be carried out at any time.
2. Muscle relaxation is not as necessary for elbow joint arthroscopy as compared with other small joint arthroscopy.
3. Functional observations can be made.

Therefore, anesthesias other than intraarticular should be reserved for those cases where surgery is to be performed.

Preparation and Positioning of the Patient

The patient undresses in the surgical anteroom. Arthroscopy is carried out with the patient on the operating table, lying supine or side, as required for each approach. The supine position is useful for supracondylar approaches, and the side position is useful for radial and supraolecranon approaches. The position of the elbow must be also changed for each approach, with the forearm supported by an assistant.

Disinfection is made from the upper arm to the finger tips, the same as for an elbow joint operation. Then a sterile stocking is placed over the upper limb.

Photography

The arthroscope is attached to the camera by an adaptor designed by the author. Color photographs, 14 mm in diameter, can be taken with an exposure time of one eighth to one thirtieth of a second using Ektachrome (EL) film (ASA 400).

Punch Biopsy

The punch biopsy of villi or similar tissues is conducted blindly through the same outer sheath after removing the arthroscope. In some cases, punch biopsy during arthroscopy may be carried out by introducing the punch from another site of insertion.

SYSTEMATIC OBSERVATION OF THE ELBOW JOINT USING THE POSTERIOR RADIAL APPROACH (Figs. 88–93)

The patient is put in the lateral position on his normal side with the elbow joint flexed at 90° and the forearm pronated. After making a stab skin incision at the insertion point, the outer sheath with the sharp trocar is inserted in an anteromedial direction toward the humeroradial joint space through the posterior fibers of the lateral collateral ligament. The capsular puncture is performed by placing the blunt trocar in the outer sheath and rotating the instrument. With the elbow joint flexed at 30° and the forearm supinated, the instrument is further inserted until the tip of the blunt trocar reaches the lateral facet of the trochlear notch. Then the blunt trocar is pushed into the medial pouch beyond the central eminence of the trochlear notch. The blunt trocar is then exchanged for the arthroscope. On looking through the scope, the inner surface of the capsule is yellowish-white and small vessels are seen. Large amount of villi in various sizes and forms can be inspected. By withdrawing the arthroscope, the central eminence, the trochlear groove, and the lateral facet of the trochlear notch can be observed. The eminence and the lateral facet are white and glossy, but the groove looks slightly yellowish-white and less glossy. Also, the transverse sulcus of the trochlear notch is found to be yellowish to reddish and of varying shape. By further withdrawing the arthroscope, the humeroradial interspace can be examined. The humeral capitulum looks spherical, white, and glossy. The radial fovea is also flat and glossy, but is slightly yellowish-white. Occasionally the circumferential synovial fluid, which is usually clear and spinnable, and the small vessels are seen. However, for inspection of these regions, the anteromedial supracondylar approach is more suitable. In these two interspaces, the functional examination can be made by moving the elbow joint and rotating the forearm.

After the arthroscope is exchanged for the blunt trocar, and with the joint flexed at 100° and the forearm pronated, the trocar is entered in a posteromedial direction toward the

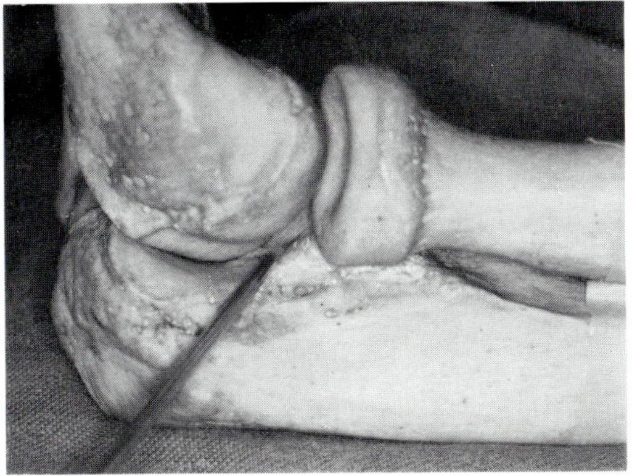

Fig. 88 Humeroradial interspace.

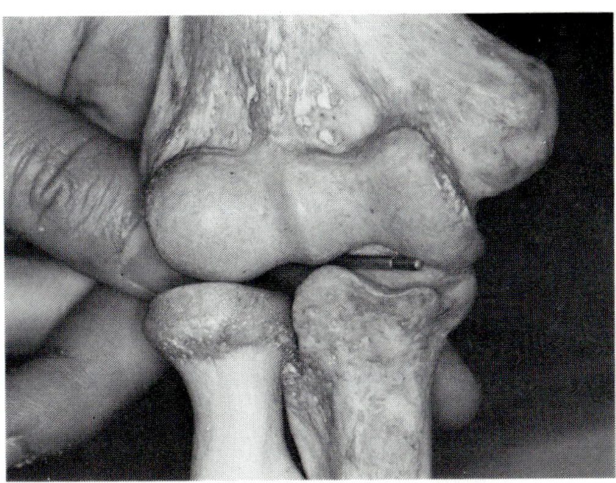

Fig. 89 Humeroulnar interspace.

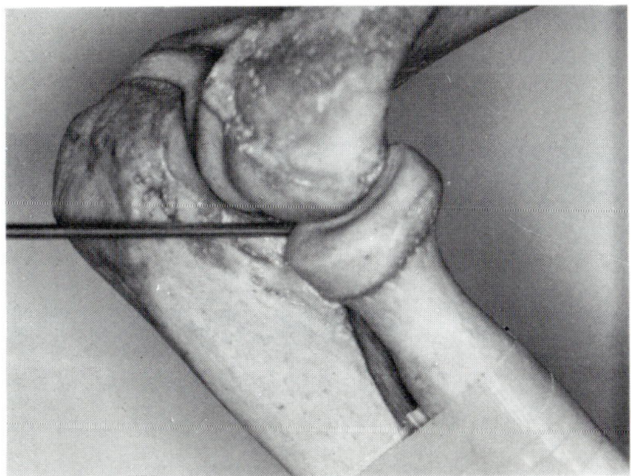

Fig. 90 Proximal radioulnar interspace.

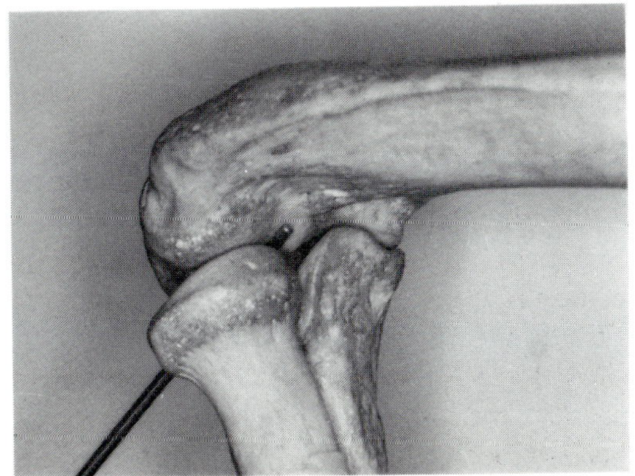

Fig. 91 Radial fossa.

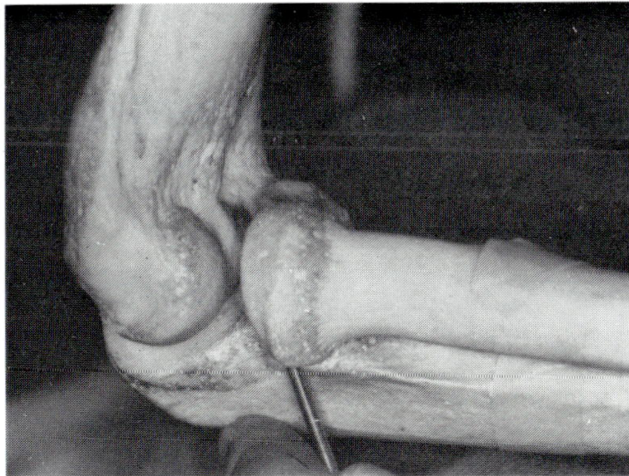

Fig. 92 Coronoid fossa.

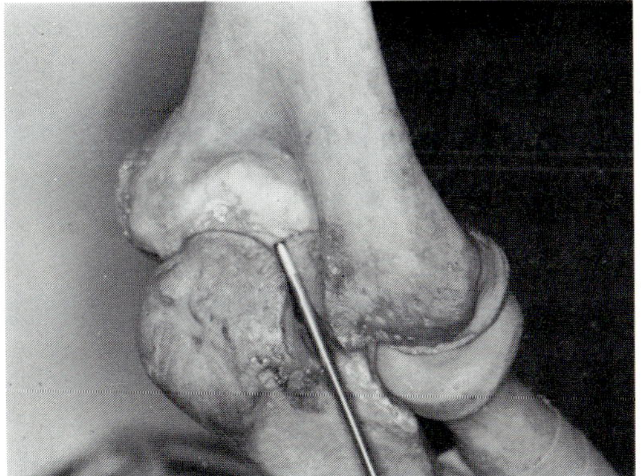

Fig. 93 Olecranon fossa.

proximal radioulnar joint. Next, while extending the joint to 60°, the blunt trocar is directed posterolaterally and the tip of it is pushed into the space between the articular surfaces of the radial annular ligament. The radial notch looks white and glossy, and the articular circumference of the radius head is the same, but the inner surface of the annular ligament looks yellow, less glossy, and plicate.

For inspection of these regions, detailed findings can be obtained by using supracondylar approaches. They show the tongue-like fat pad overlying the proximal radioulnar joint. Occasionally these maneuvers are obstructed by the ridge formation around the radial fovea or by the large circumferential synovial fold.

After observation of these regions, the instrument with the blunt trocar is introduced in an anteromedial direction, with the elbow joint flexed at 100°, into the radial fossa and coronoid fossa. Next, the instrument is pushed in a posterior direction into the olecranon fossa with the joint flexed at 45°. The capsule, villi, fat pads, and articular cartilage can be inspected in these three regions. To inspect the tip of the coronoid fossa, the anteromedial supracondylar approach should be used. To inspect the olecranon fossa and the tip of the olecranon, the posteromedial supraolecranal approach should be used. For inspection of the lateral pouch, the anterior radial approach and the supracondylar approaches are more suitable.

OBSERVATION OF THE ELBOW JOINT USING OTHER APPROACHES

Anterior Radial Approach

With the patient in a lateral position, and the elbow flexed at 90°, the trocar is inserted at right angles to the skin between the humeral capitulum and the radius head, and entered between the articular surfaces of the humeroradial joint with the aid of the obturator puncture of the joint. The trocar is then moved inside to reach the medial pouch across the central eminence of the trochlear notch. After examination of the medial pouch, the scope is retracted for inspection of the lateral interspace of the humeroulnar joint. It is then replaced with the obturator and the elbow joint is bent to 100°. The trocar reaches the coronoid fossa when it is advanced in an anteromedial direction. If the trocar is advanced in a posteromedial direction while extending the elbow joint, it will reach the olecranon fossa. With this approach, the radial fossa, the coronoid fossa, the humeroradial interspace, and the lateral part of the humeroulnar interspace can be observed.

Anterolateral Supracondylar Approach

The patient is put in a supine position and the elbow joint is flexed to 30°. The trocar is inserted into the skin at a right angle about two fingerbreadth from the tip of the lateral epicondyle of the humerus. It is advanced along the anterior surface of the humerus, and then directed posteromedially into the radial fossa. Next, the elbow joint is flexed to 45° and the trocar is advanced to the humeroradial joint. At this point, the lateral pouch, the superior aspect of the proximal radioulnar interspace, the superior aspect of the radioannular interspace, the radial fovea, and the radial fossa can be examined. The functional observation of both the radioannular interspace and the proximal radioulnar interspace can be carried out by rotation of the forearm. This approach may be used for detailed observation of the anterolateral part of the joint cavity.

Anteromedial Supracondylar Approach

The patient is put in a supine position and the elbow joint is flexed to 45°. The trocar is inserted into the skin at a right angle about one and a half fingerbreadth from the tip of the medial epicondyle of the humerus. The obturator is placed along the anterior surface of the humerus, and the trocar is advanced to the coronoid fossa almost parallel to the forearm. It is then inserted into the joint cavity. The elbow joint is then flexed to 80° and the trocar is advanced in a posterolateral direction toward the humeroradial interspace and the lateral synovial pouch.

In these space, movement of the scope is relatively free and rotation of the forearm is also free. The examiner can make functional observations of the proximal radioulnar interspace and the radioannular interspace. The scope is then retracted to the coronoid fossa and observation of the coronoid process tip and the anterior third of the humeroulnar interspace is carried out. This approach is used for observation of the lateral pouch, the coronoid fossa, the coronoid process, the anterior third of the humeroulnar interspace, and also for functional examination of the proximal radioulnar interspace and the radioannular interspace.

Posterolateral Supraolecranal Approach

The patient is put in a lateral position. The elbow joint is flexed to 60° and the trocar is inserted into the skin at a right angle about two fingerbreadth from the tip of the proximal end of the olecranon and just lateral of the triceps muscle. The tip of the obturator is placed along the posterior surface of the humerus, and the trocar is advanced in an anteromedial direction. It is then inserted into the olecranon fossa.

Posteromedial Supraolecranal Approach

The patient is put in a lateral position. The elbow joint is flexed to 90°. The trocar is inserted into the skin at a right angle about two fingerbreadth from the center of the proximal end of the olecranon and just medial of the triceps muscle. The tip of obturator is placed along the humerus, and, while protecting the ulnar nerve with the examiner's fingers, the trocar is advanced laterally and inserted into the olecranon fossa. Both approaches of the above procedure are used for examination of the olecranon fossa, the tip of the olecranon, and the posterior fourth of the humeroulnar interspace. However, because there are many villi in the olecranon fossa, sufficient saline solution or gas should be injected before observation. Movement of the scope in this cavity and also in the elbow joint is severely limited.

NORMAL ARTHROSCOPIC VIEWS AND THE SELECTION OF APPROACHES

Observation of a normal elbow joint is made on the regions indicated in Figure 80. These regions are also listed in Table 12. These regions cannot all be examined by a single puncture procedure. The arthroscopic view of each approach reveals certain dead spaces because of the anatomic complexity of the humeroulnar joint. One third of the central region of the humeroulnar interspace and the sacciform recess cannot be examined by any approach. The posterior radial and anterior radial approaches are suitable for routine arthroscopic examinations of the elbow joint. The anterolateral supracondylar approach allows observation of the anterior compartment of the joint cavity. The anteromedial supracondylar approach is suitable for examination of one third of the anterior part of the trochlea, anterior one third of the front of the trochlear notch, the tip of the coronoid process, and synovial villi in the coronoid fossa. To observe the region of the posterior third of the trochlea, the region of the posterior fourth of the trochlear notch, and the tip of the olecranon, supraolecranal approaches are suitable. In particular, the posterolateral supraolecranal approach is suitable for observation of the posterior region of the lateral concave facet of the trochlear notch, and the posteromedial supraolecranal approach is suitable for observation of the posterior region of the medial concave facet of the trochlear notch.

The lateral facet of the trochlea looks white, glossy, and smooth. The trochlear groove is less glossy and has a somewhat yellowish-white color, but looks smooth. The medial

Table 12 Selection of approaches in elbow joint arthroscopy

Anatomic detail examined	Approach					
	Anterior radial	Transligamentous posterior radial	Anterolateral supracondylar	Anteromedial supracondylar	Posterolateral supraolecranal	Posteromedial supraolecranal
Humeroradial interspace	++	++	++	++	—	—
Radioannular interspace	+	++	++	++	—	—
Proximal radioulnar interspace	+	++	++	++	—	—
Medial humeroulnar interspace	—	—	—	(+) ant.	—	(+) post.
Lateral humeroulnar interspace	++	++	(+) ant.	—	(+) post.	(+) post.
Medial synovial pouch	(+) ant.	(+) mid. ant.	—	(+) ant.	—	—
Lateral synovial pouch	++	+	++	++	—	—
Radial fossa	++	++	++	—	—	—
Coronoid fossa	+	++	—	++	—	—
Olecranon fossa	—	+	—	—	++	++
Sacciform recess	—	—	—	—	—	—
Humeral capitulum	++	++	(+) ant.	(+) mid.	(+) post.	(+) post.
Radial fovea	++	++	++	++	—	—
Articular circumference (radius)	+	++	++	+	—	—
Annular ligament	+	++	++	+	—	—
Radial notch (ulna)	+	++	+	—	—	—
Medial convex facet (trochlea)	+	—	—	(+) ant.	(+) post.	(+) post.
Lateral convex facet (trochlea)	+	++	(+) ant.	(+) ant. mid.	(+) post.	(+) post.
Trochlear groove	+	++	(+) ant.	(+) ant. mid.	(+) post.	(+) post.
Medial concave facet (trochlear notch)	—	—	—	(+) ant.	—	(+) post.
Lateral concave facet (trochlear notch)	++	++	(+) ant.	(+) ant. mid.	(+) lat.	(+) mid.
Coronoid process	+	+	(+) lat.	++	—	—
Olecranon	+	+	—	—	++	++

++ = Suitable. + = Possible. — = Impossible. (+) = Partially possible. ant. = Anterior part only. mid. = Middle part only. post. = Posterior part only. lat. = Lateral part only.

facet of the trochlea looks less glossy and more yellowish in color. The lateral facet of the trochlear notch looks white in color, glossy, and smooth, but the transverse sulcus of the trochlear notch has individual variations. It reveals various forms and sizes ranging from a band-form impression type to a fibrillation type of articular cartilage. The medial facet of the trochlear notch looks white and less glossy, and occasionally a fibrillation of joint cartilage will be found. The tip of the coronoid process and the olecranon look white in color and glossy, but villi frequently block the visual field.

To observe the surface of the humeral capitulum and radius head, the posterior radial approach is suitable and makes it possible to observe almost the whole area. With the anterior radial approach, the posterior one-third area of the humeral capitulum cannot be observed. The anterolateral supracondylar approach permits viewing of the anterior third. The humeral capitulum looks global in shape, and has a white, glossy, and smooth appearance. However, the color of tissue becomes yellow and less glossy with aging. The surface of the radius head and the depression look white and smooth, but less glossy, and the peripheral eminence has a glossy appearance. With aging, the depression becomes wider, the eminence disappears, and there is fibrillation of the cartilage. The circumferential synovial fold shows wide individual variations of form and size, ranging from the ring-shaped type to the type that covers the whole area of the radial head surface. Occasionally a large quantity of villi is also found.

For observation of the proximal radioulnar interspace, the posterior radial approach and the anterolateral supracondylar approach are suitable. The tongue-like fat pad found in this space can be also observed by the anterior radial and anteromedial supracondylar approaches.

The radial notch of the ulna can be observed by the posterior radial approach and anterolateral supracondylar approach. The radial notch looks white, smooth, and glossy in a young patient, but in older patients it shows a yellowish, less glossy appearance, with fibrillation and joint cartilage deficiency. These two approaches are both similarly suitable for the radioannular interspace.

However, the anteromedial supracondylar approach is most suitable for functional observations of this joint-like space. The circumferential surface of the radius head looks smooth, white, and glossy, but the annular ligament surface presents a yellowish-white and less glossy appearance. It frequently has a circular fold. In the case of an elbow that has a relatively large circumferential synovial fold and a ridge on the peripheral margin of the radius head that has been formed through aging, satisfactory observation cannot be achieved. The tongue-like fat pad varies in appearance, and is sometimes squeezed into the proximal radioulnar interspace, making observation difficult. With the supracondylar approach and posterior radial approach, the central part of the medial pouch can be investigated. The anterior radial approach permits observation of the anterior region. The posteromedial supraolecranal approach can be used for observation of the posterior region, but is insufficient for complete observation. The synovial wall looks yellowish-white and the small blood vessels can be seen clearly. The synovial villi have various shapes ranging from slender to nodular, and the quantity of villi also varies with each individual. The results of the examination are very similar to those of the medial pouch examination.

Observation of the sacciform recess is a very difficult procedure. The anterior radial approach is more suitable for the radial fossa, but the anterolateral supracondylar and posterior radial approaches can also be applied. The anteromedial supracondylar approach is the most suitable approach for coronoid fossa examination, but the anterior radial and posterior radial approaches are also suitable.

The supraolecranal approach can be used for olecranon fossa examination, and radial approaches provide lateral views of the observation. In the radial, coronoid and sacciform fossae, a large yellowish fat pad with villi attached to the capsular ligament can be seen. Because a large quantity of villi always inhibits the visual field, caution is needed when applying the pressurized saline injection for the examination.

CLINICAL CASES

Typical arthroscopic views of the pathological changes are described.

Synovial Membrane and Synovial Folds

The precise appearance of these synovial tissues is determined by arthroscopy. There are many different types of synovial folds. The arthroscopic diagnosis of arthritis is the same as in knee joint arthroscopy. In the case of rheumatoid arthritis, a large amount of villi are seen in the lateral synovial pouch. In the case of advanced osteoarthritis, a large amount of villi can be observed in the olecranon fossa. With an infection, a large quantity of nodular-shaped villi fill the whole area of the joint cavity.

Articular cartilage

The appearance of articular cratilage changes to yellow and is less glossy with aging. Occasionally, fibrillation, ulceration, and disappearance of the cartilage are found. In the case of osteoarthritis, these changes are observed mainly in the radial fovea, and also in the proximal radioulnar interspace. In trauma, fracture lines and bruises on the cartilage of the lateral facet of the trochlear notch can frequently be observed. However, these changes should be differentiated from those caused by degeneration.

Other Disorders

Loose bodies can occasionally be found in the olecranon fossa. In the case of osteochondritis dissecans, the olecranon fossa should be examined carefully with arthroscopy, and the same care should be taken to inspect the humeral capitulum.

Table 13 Clinical cases (January 1975 to December 1979)

Total number of patients	201
Males	109
Females	92
Age	5–79 years (average, 45)
Total number of joints examined	213
Right elbow joints	107
Left elbow joints	94
Both elbow joints	12 (6 cases)
Diseases	
Osteoarthritis	97
Rheumatoid arthritis	95
Suppurative arthritis	7
Traumatic arthritis	10
Others	4

CASES EXAMINED

From January 1975 to December 1979, 213 elbow joints in 201 patients were arthroscopically examined, as summarized in Table 13. No cases with side effects such as postoperative infection or joint blood tumor were experienced.

Changes in synovial villi and interarticular cartilage were about the same as observed in the knee joint arthroscopy, but the observation of elbow joints indicated localization of the diseased part, depending on the type of disease. The typical arthroscopic findings of the respective diseases are described.

Osteoarthritis

The cases of osteoarthritis can be roughly divided into two groups: (1) those complaining of gradual articular contracture, as seen in relatively young people who play such sports as baseball and tennis, and articular contracture with an external injury suffered in the past; and (2) articular contracture and articular dropsy seen in patients who are engaged in agriculture, forestry, and other similar jobs.

The synovial villi are of the slender type with few blood vessels observed growing in olecranon fossa or lateral joint cavity wall. The articular cartilage shows characteristic changes. In the first group, a sprain on the articular cartilage is observed in such parts as the radial fossa, humeroulnar interspace, and radioulnar proximal interspace, with a torn cartilage piece incarcerated into the joint interspace in many cases. The articular cartilage area other than the diseased part is in relatively good condition.

In the second group, the articular cartilage over almost the entire area is affected. Especially noticeable are the formation of osteophyte in the lateral marginal zone of radial fovea, and the destructive degeneration in the radioulnar proximal interspace and medial humeroulnar interspace. Also, joint mice are present in some cases (Figs. 94–97).

Rheumatoid Arthritis

In cases of rheumatoid arthritis at a relatively early stage, villi in various forms with rich blood vessels grow thickly all over the joint cavity—especially in the lateral joint cavity wall and the circumferential synovial fold. Mainly in the articular cartilage, the synovial membrane is observed extending from the marginal zone of the cartilage. In some cases an advanced stage, the joint interspace is filled with thickly grown villi. In other cases, the synovial membrane grows markedly thick with decreased villi. The articular cartilage indicates destructive degeneration all over the area (Figs. 98–103).

Suppurative Arthritis

In acute suppurative arthritis cases, villi with rich blood vessels grow thickly over the entire joint cavity, with many suspensions and necrotic tissue. The articular cartilage surface remains normal in many cases. In advanced cases, the articular cartilage surface, too, is destroyed and hard to distinguish from other diseases (Figs. 104–106).

Joint Mice

Joint mice (loose bodies) are very often combined with osteoarthritis and observed in the olecranon fossa and lateral joint cavity (Figs. 107–110).

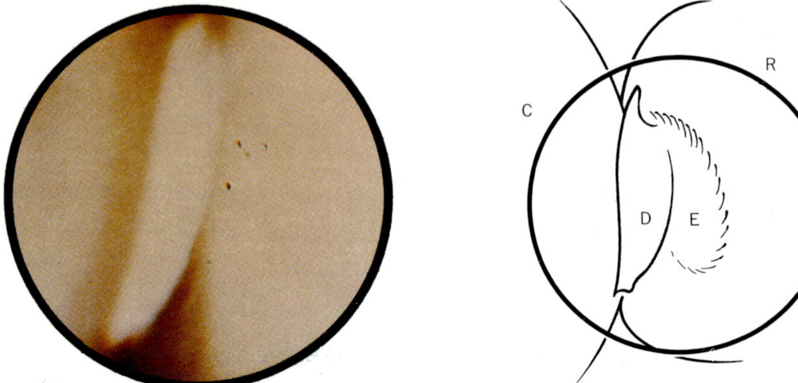

Fig. 94 Case 1. A 23-year-old man with osteoarthritis, humeroradial joint interspace of right elbow. Transligamentous posterior radial approach. No injury suffered in the past. Played baseball for many years. Main complaint: articular contracture. Erosion (E) observed in radial fovea with torn cartilage piece (D) extending into the humeroradial joint interspace. (C) Humeral capitulum, (R) Radial fovea.

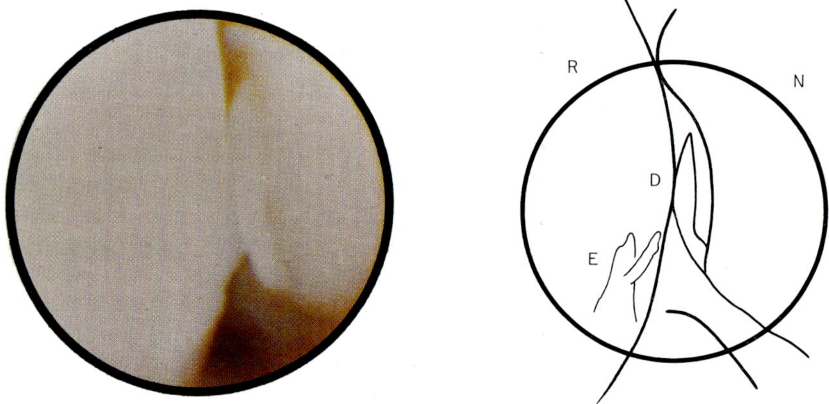

Fig. 95 Case 2. An 18-year-old man with osteoarthritis, radioulnar joint interspace of left elbow. Anteromedial supracondylar approach. No past injury suffered. Played baseball for many years. Complained chiefly of pain in the elbow joint on movement and difficulty in turning the forearm. The torn cartilage piece (D) can be seen on the radius notch. Also, erosion (E) observed in the radial fovea. (R) Radial fovea. (N) Radial notch of the ulna.

Injuries

Different types of damage to the articular cartilage surface are observed, depending on the nature and degree of the injury suffered (Fig. 111).

Other Disorders

Osteochondritis dissecans, synovial osteochondromatosis, and other disorders present characteristic arthroscopic images (Fig. 112).

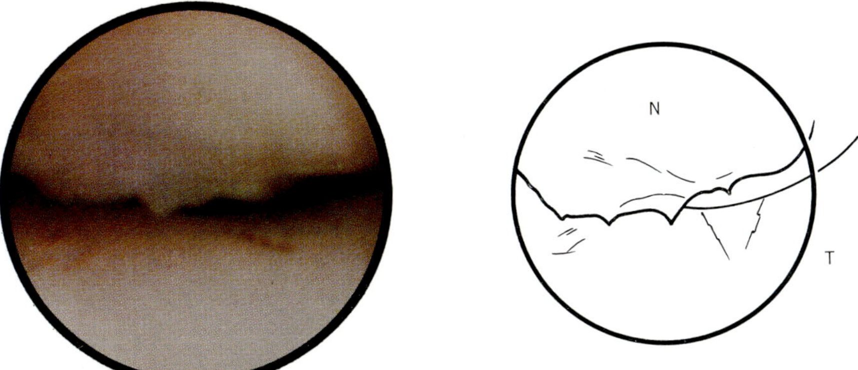

Fig. 96 Case 3. A 39-year-old man with osteoarthritis, the anterior part of humeroulnar joint of right elbow. Anteromedial supracondylar approach. Patient suffered a fracture of olecranon in the past. Main complaint: limited bending of the elbow joint. The facet (N) inside the trochlear notch is irregular with degeneration observed on the facet inside the trochlea (T).

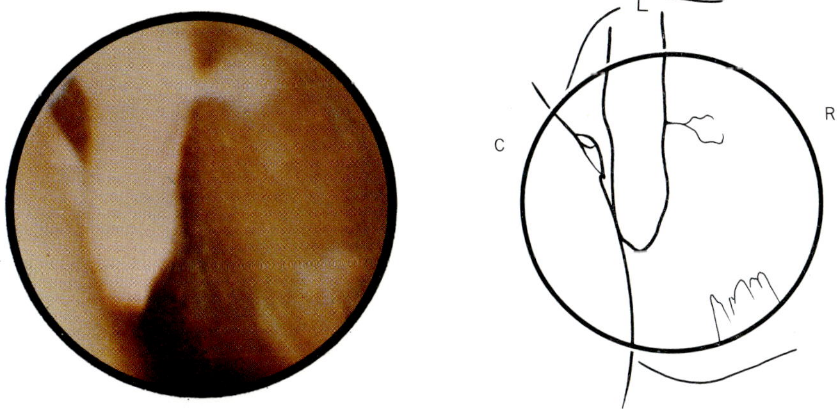

Fig. 97 Case 4. A 58-year-old man with osteoarthritis, the humeroradial joint interspace of right elbow. Transligamentous posterior radial approach. No injury suffered in past. Engaged in agriculture for many years. Main complaint: contracture of elbow joint. Humeral capitulum (C) is in relatively good condition, but the articular cartilage of radial fovea (R) is destroyed and lost. Loose bodies (L) are observed in the interspace.

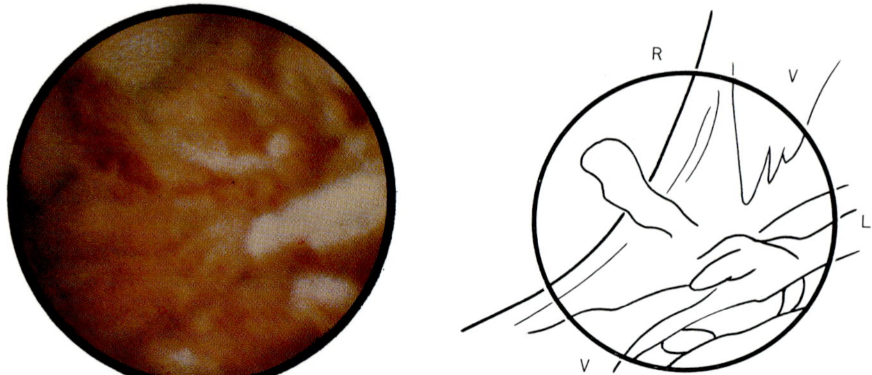

Fig. 98 Case 5. A 34-year-old woman with rheumatoid arthritis, lateral synovial pouch of right elbow. Anteromedial supracondylar approach. Radial fovea (R) is relatively normal. Villi (V) have grown thickly on the inside surface of the lateral synovial pouch. (L) Loose bodies.

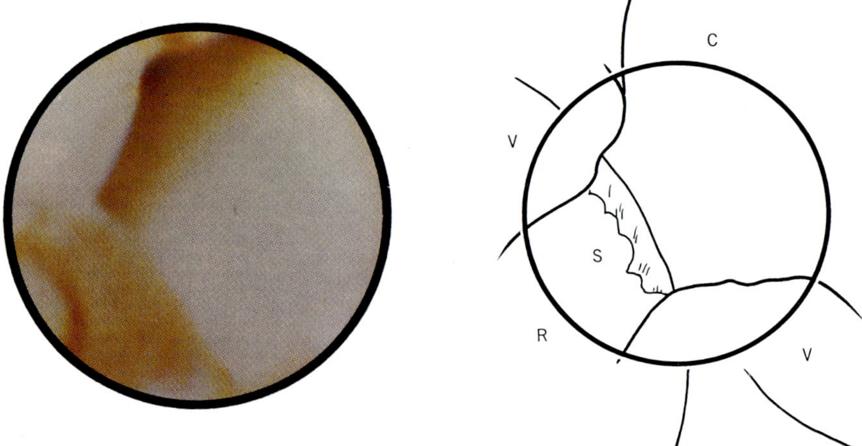

Fig. 99 Case 6. A 35-year-old woman with rheumatoid arthritis, humeroradial joint interspace of left elbow. Transligamentous posterior radial approach. Humeral capitulum (C) is normal. Synovial membrane (S) is seen extruding into radial fovea (R), with villi growing thickly. (V) Villi.

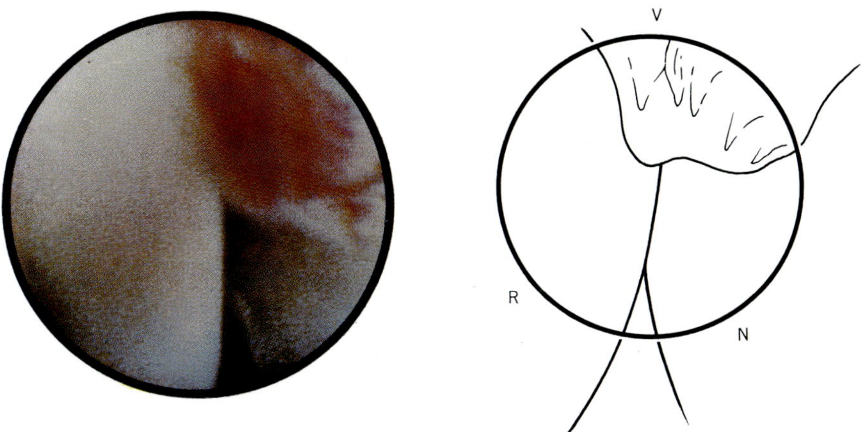

Fig. 100 Case 7. An 18-year-old girl with rheumatoid arthritis, radioulnar promixal interspace of left elbow. Anterolateral supracondylar approach. Radial fovea (R) and radial notch (N) remain normal. The tongue-like fat pad has thickened, with rich blood vessels and villi (V) growing thickly.

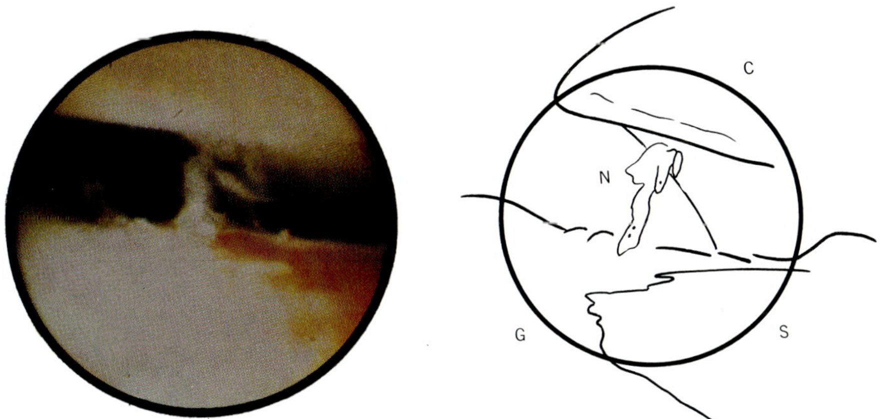

Fig. 101 Case 8. A 24-year-old woman with rheumatoid arthritis, coronoid fossa of left elbow. Anteromedial supracondylar approach. Coronoid fossa (C) is normal. Synovial membrane (S) is observed invading into the anterior surface of trochlea (G), with some necrotic tissues (N).

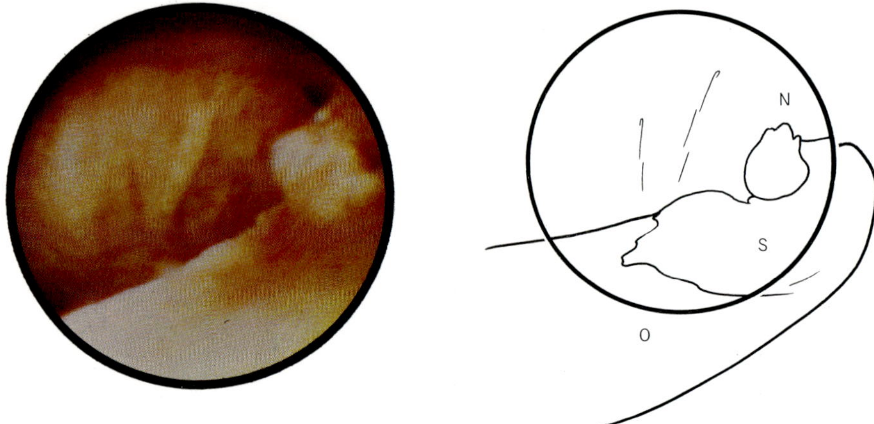

Fig. 102 Case 9. A 48-year-old woman with rheumatoid arthritis, olecranon fossa of left elbow. Transligamentous posterior radial approach. Synovial membrane (S) is seen intruding into the tip of olecranon (O) with some necrotic tissues (N). No villi are found growing.

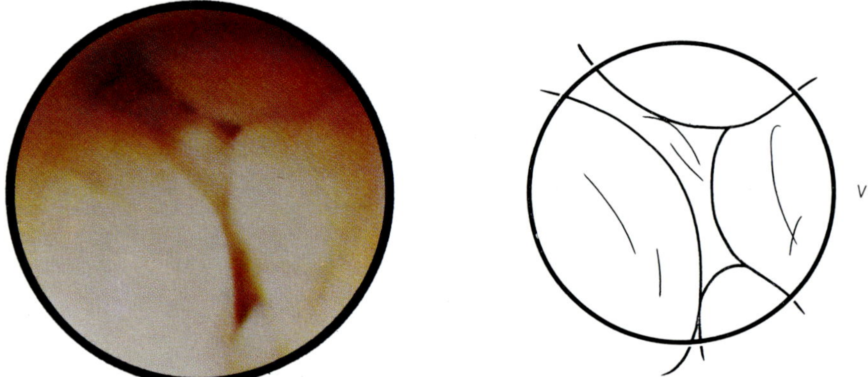

Fig. 103 Case 10. A 38-year-old woman with rheumatoid arthritis, the humeroradial joint interspace of left elbow. Transligamentous posterior radial approach. The interspace is filled up with villi (V) growing in the form of knots. No cartilaginous surface is observed.

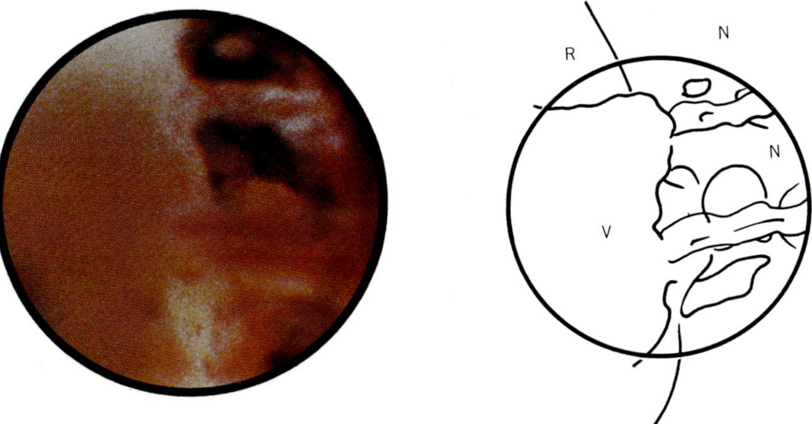

Fig. 104 Case 11. A 30-year-old woman with suppurative arthritis, the lateral synovial pouch of right elbow. Anterolateral supracondylar approach. The radial fovea (R) is covered with grown villi (V) and necrotic tissues (N) are also observed.

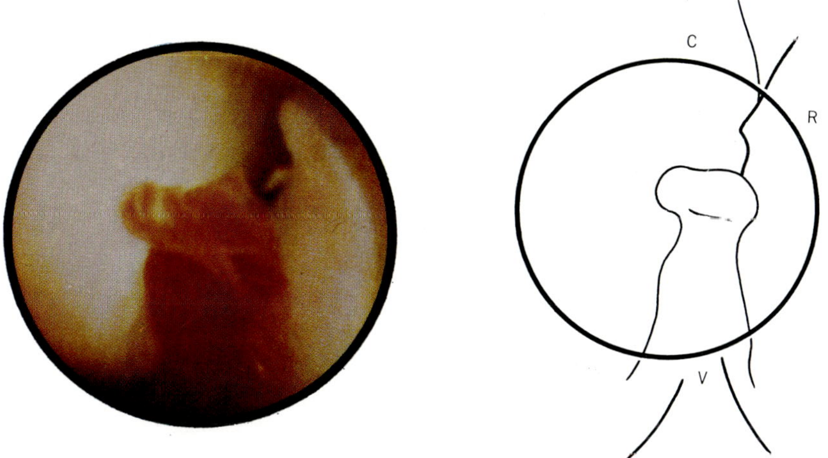

Fig. 105 Case 12. A 33-year-old woman with suppurative arthritis, the humeroradial joint interspace of right elbow. Transligamentous posterior radial approach. The capitulum (C) and radial fovea (R) have lost luster and degenerated slightly. Villi (V) with rich blood vessels are invading into the interspace.

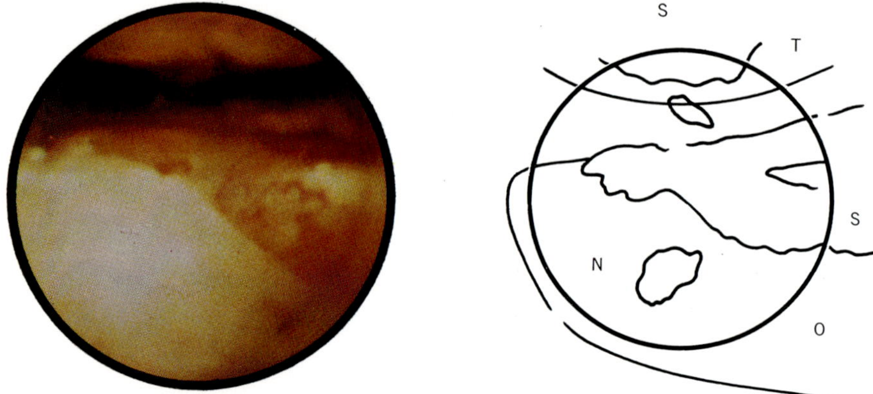

Fig. 106 Case 13. A 39-year-old man with suppurative arthritis, the posterior part of radio-ulnar joint interspace of right elbow. Transligamentous posterior radial approach. The lateral facet of trochlea (T) and the lateral facet in the posterior part of trochlear notch (O) are both destroyed markedly and covered with synovial membrane (S). Also, necrotic tissues (N) are observed.

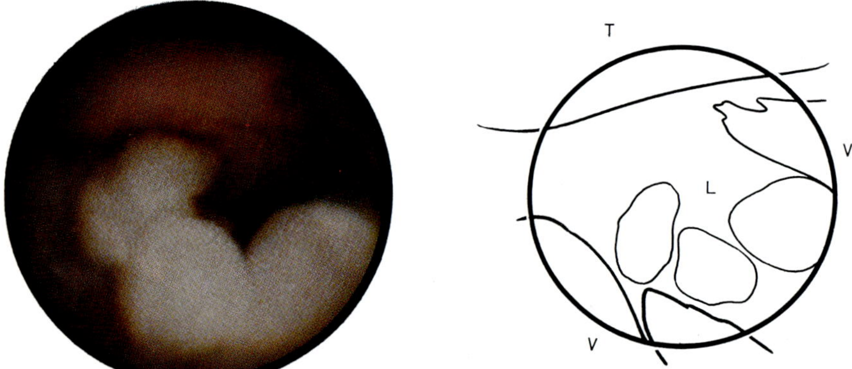

Fig. 107 Case 14. A 68-year-old man with loose bodies, olecranon fossa of right elbow. Posteromedial supraolecranal approach. Villi (V) are not thickly grown. Three loose bodies (L) are observed on the posterior part of trochlea (T).

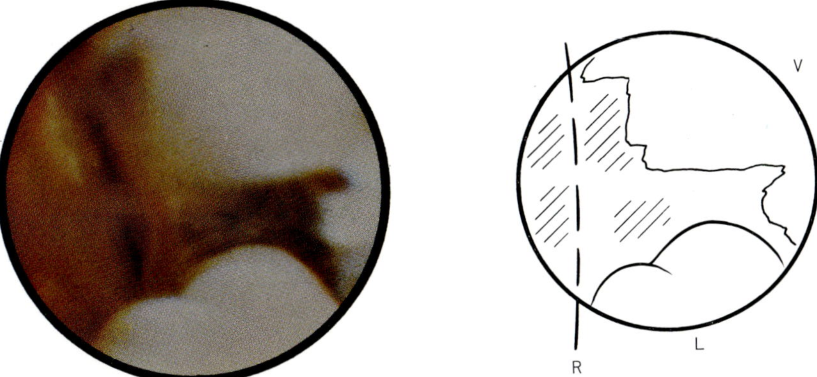

Fig. 108 Case 15. A 45-year-old man with loose bodies, lateral joint pouch cavity of right elbow. Anterolateral supracondylar approach. Thickly grown villi (V) and a large loose body (L) are present. The loose body is interrupted into the humeroradial joint interspace, combined with an injury in the radial fovea (R).

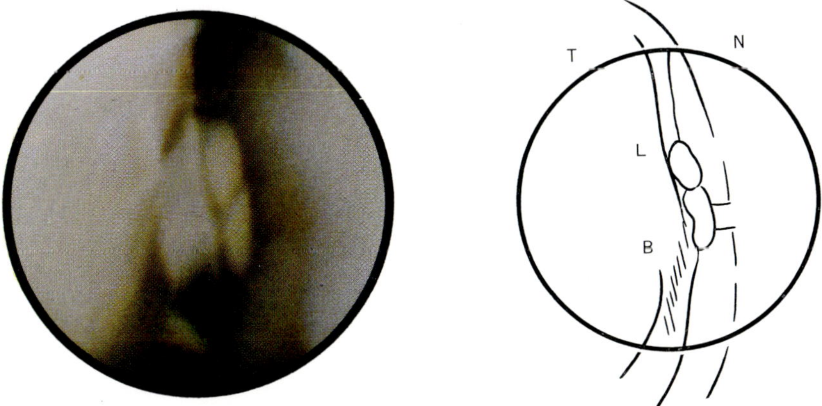

Fig. 109 Case 16. A 33-year-old man with loose bodies, central part of the radioulnar joint interspace of right elbow. Transligamentous posteroradial approach. The trochlear notch of ulna (N) is normal, but ulceration (B) is observed in the cartilaginous surface of the trochlea of the humerous (T). The loose bodies (L) interrupt into the interspace.

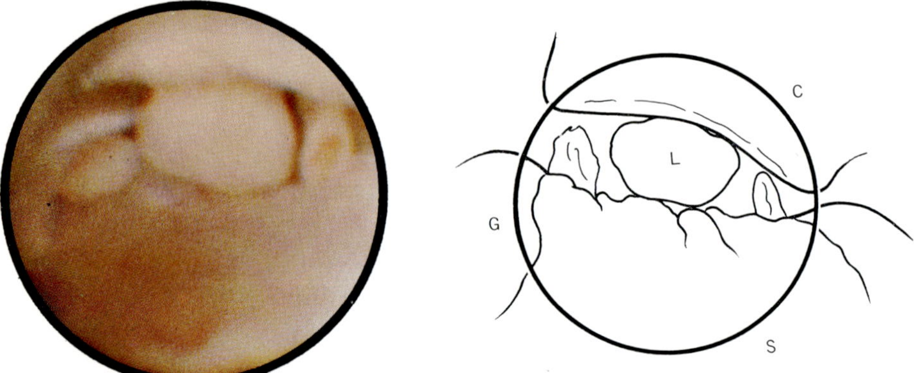

Fig. 110 Case 17. A 65-year-old man with loose bodies, coronoid fossa of left elbow. Anteromedial supracondylar approach. The coronoid fossa (C) remains normal, but the anterior surface of the trochlear sulcus (G) is covered with synovial membrane (S) and the loose bodies (L) is contained within the interspace. This loose body is seen as a complication to rheumatoid arthritis.

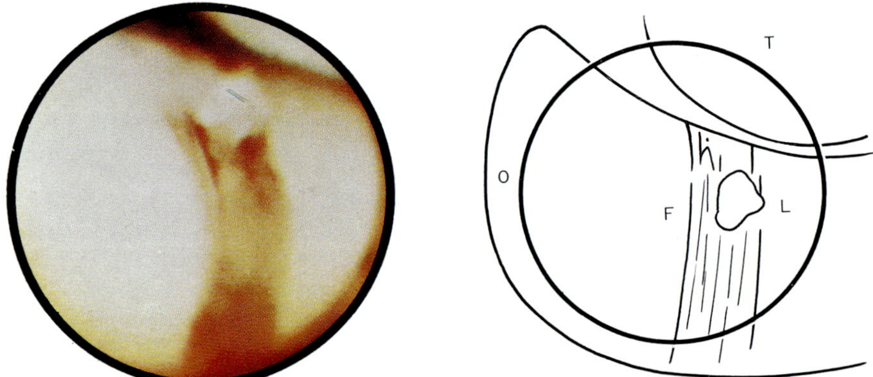

Fig. 111 Case 18. A 28-year-old man with a fracture of olecranon, the posterior part of the humeroulnar joint interspace of right elbow. Transligamentous posterior radial approach. No damage is observed in the trochlea (T). A fracture, bleeding (F), and torn cartilage pieces (L) are observed in the posterior part of the lateral facet of the trochlear notch (O).

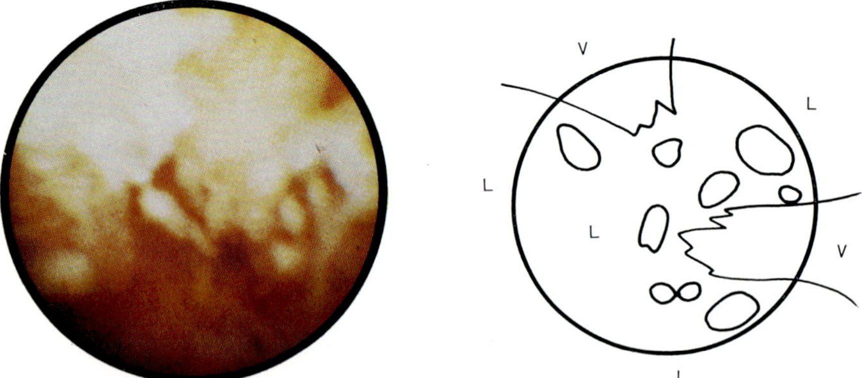

Fig. 112 Case 19. A 48-year-old woman with osteochondromatosis, left elbow, olecranon fossa. Posterolateral supraolecranal approach. While no thickly grown villi (V) are observed, many loose bodies (L) are seen sticking to the capsular membrane.

6

Arthroscopy of the Wrist Joint

Arthroscopy of the wrist joint was performed in 32 clinical cases and three amputated arms. The findings were compared with findings in 11 dissected wrists (four cadavers and three amputated arms).

Among the clinical cases were 29 cases of rheumatoid arthritis, one case of fracture of the distal ulna, one case of fracture of the lunate bone and one case of chondromalacia of the lunate bone (Table 14).

ARTHROSCOPIC ANATOMY OF THE WRIST JOINT

The wrist joint (Fig. 113) is formed by the distal ends of the radius and ulna and the proximal row of carpal bones (scaphoid, lunate, and triangular bones). The distal end of the radius is rectangular and concave and is divided into two parts by a smooth dorsovolar ridge. The radial portion articulates with the scaphoid bone, and the ulnar portion with the lunate bone.

A round or ovoid articular disk is located at the distal end of the ulna, and it may have a central or an eccentric hole permitting communication of the radiocarpal joint cavity with the distal radioulnar joint. The proximal row of carpal bones is convex and is connected with the intercarpal ligaments. The wrist joint is surrounded by a capsule and strengthened by the radiocarpal (dorsal and volar) and collateral (radial and ulnar) ligaments. There is usually a plica in the dorsal joint capsule.

Table 14 Arthroscopy of the wrist joint

Joints examined	Number	
Clinical cases*		32
Rheumatoid arthritis	29	
Fracture of lunate	1	
Fracture of distal ulna	1	
Chondromalacia of lunate	1	
Amputated limbs		2
Total		34

* Male 3, female 29.

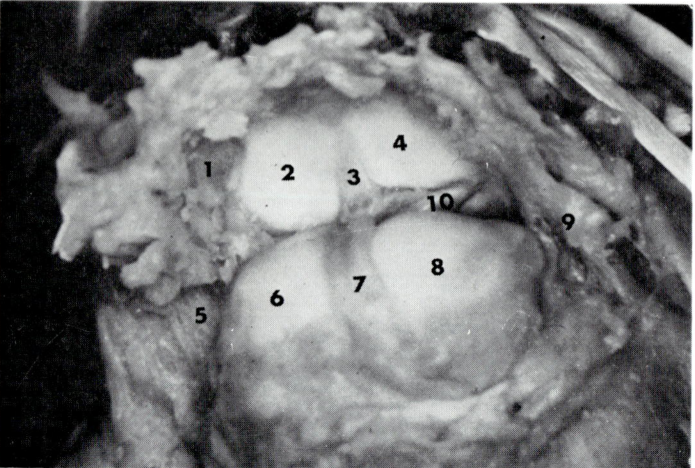

Fig. 113 Anatomic features of the right wrist joint. (1) Articular disk. (2) Radius (articular surface for lunate bone). (3) Ridge. (4) Radius (articular surface for scaphoid bone). (5) Ulnar collateral ligament. (6) Os lunatum. (7) Intercarpal ligament. (8) Os scaphoideum. (9) Radial collateral ligament. (10) Volar radiocarpal ligament.

TECHNIQUES FOR ARTHROSCOPY OF THE WRIST JOINT

The telescopes, light guide, and camera are sterilized by 24 hours exposure in a formalin vapor chamber.

Local anesthesia is adequate for arthroscopy of the wrist joint. The wrist joint is anesthetized by infiltration with 1% procaine or 1% lidocaine (Xylocaine) at the site where the arthroscope is to be inserted. The synovium may also be anesthetized by injecting 3 to 5 ml of 1% lidocaine into the joint.

Brachial block, axillary block, and general anesthesia are better for obtaining complete relaxation of the limb and a better view of the joint cavity. Use of a tourniquet at the upper arm and intravenous regional anesthesia with 10 to 15 ml of 1% lidocaine are also recommended for obtaining good muscle relaxation.

APPROACHES (Fig. 114)

Arthroscopy of the wrist joint can be carried out through dorsal approaches. A trocar puncture of the wrist joint is made at dorsal joint line, either between the extensor pollicis longus tendon and the extensor digitorum communis tendon in the dorsoradial approach, or between the extensor digitorum communis tendon and the extensor digiti quinti proprius tendon in the dorsoulnar approach.

In making a trocar puncture, the dorsal joint line of the wrist is carefully identified and the joint cavity is distended maximally with normal saline solution. With the wrist joint in a slightly volar flexed position, a small stab wound, about 2 mm, is made at the puncture site and the trocar is inserted obliquely into the dorsal joint cavity. The extensor tendons should be carefully palpated to avoid injury to the tendons. An obturator is usually used to confirm a successful puncture and for guiding the arthroscope to the desired areas in the joint cavity.

The structures seen are the dorsal joint capsule, the articular surfaces of the distal end of the radius, and the intraarticular parts of the scaphoid and lunate bones. Also seen are the intercarpal ligament, the radiocarpal (dorsal and volar) and collateral (radial and ulnar) ligaments, the articular disk, and the joint space with its fat and lining synovium. Examples are shown in Figures 115 through 124.

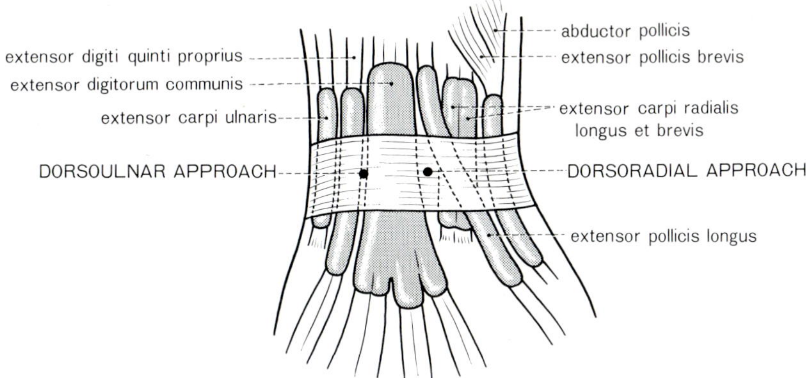

Fig. 114 Approaches of arthroscopy of wrist joint.

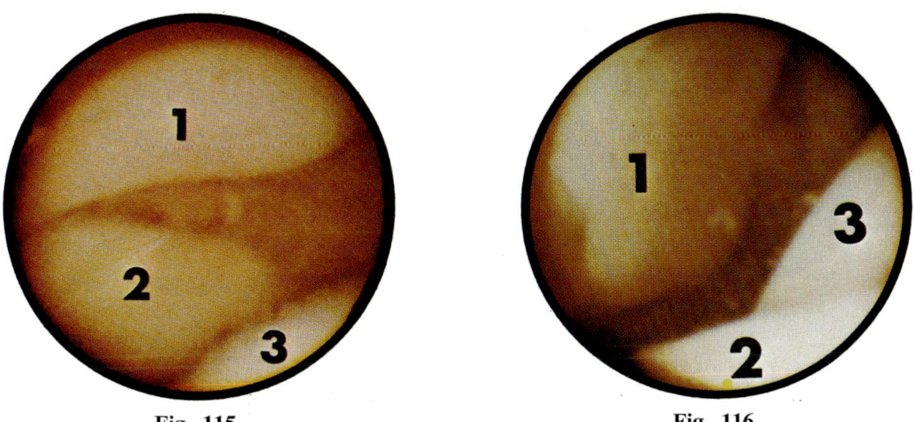

Fig. 115 **Fig. 116**

Fig. 115 Right wrist of an amputated arm, dorsoradial approach. (1) Radius. (2) Volar radiocarpal ligament. (3) Os scaphoideum.

Fig. 116 Left wrist of an amputated arm, dorsoradial approach. (1) Radius. (2) Intercarpal ligament. (3) Os lunatum.

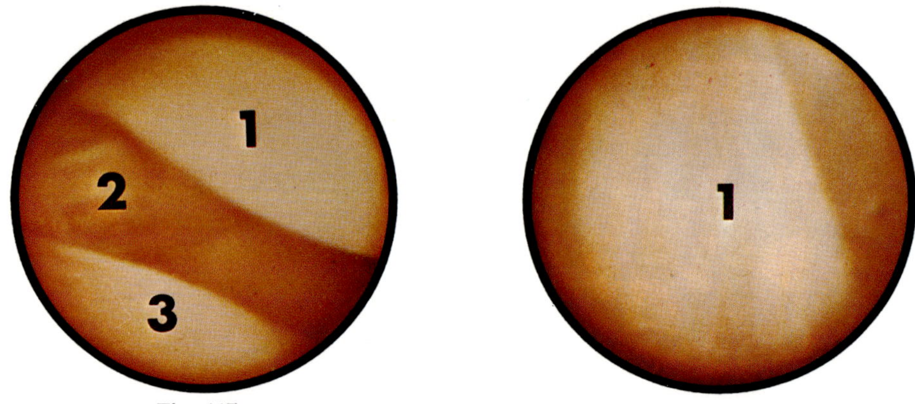

Fig. 117 Fig. 118

Fig. 117 Left wrist of an amputated arm, dorsoulnar approach. (1) Radius. (2) Volar radiocarpal ligament. (3) Os scaphoideum.

Fig. 118 Left wrist of an amputated arm, dorsoradial approach. (1) Radial collateral ligament.

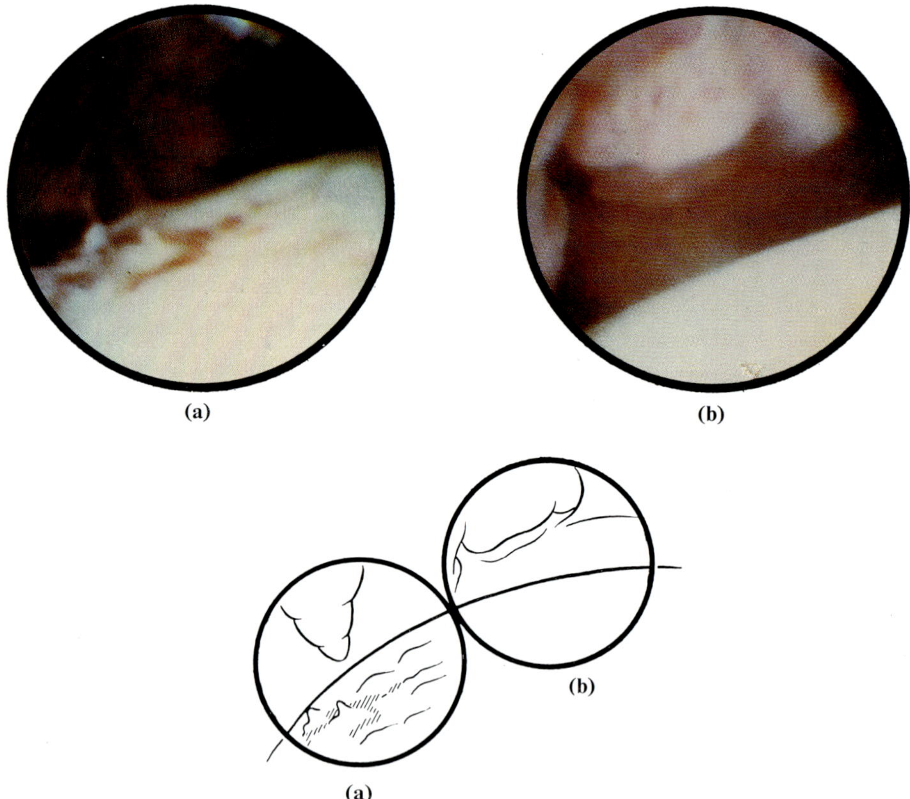

Fig. 119 A 22-year-old man with fracture of the left scaphoid. Lesions of cartilage are seen (a).

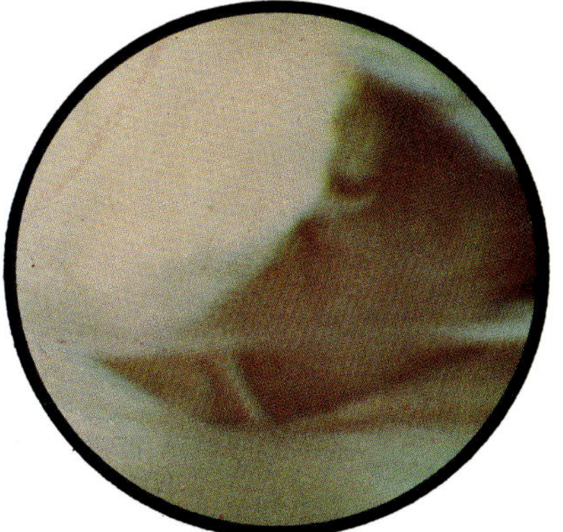

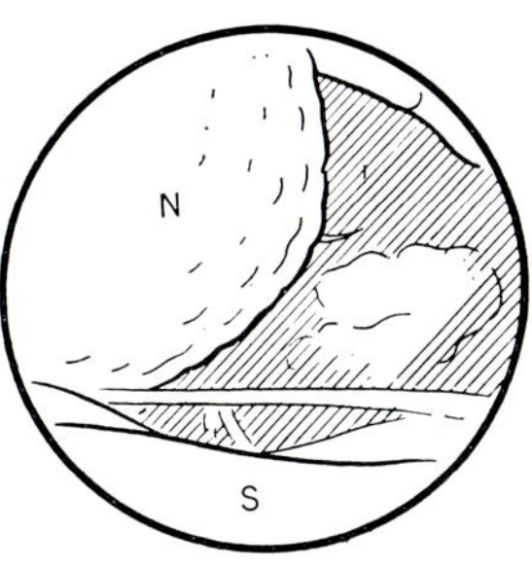

Fig. 120 A 67-year-old woman with rheumatoid arthritis of the right wrist joint. (S) Scaphoid. (N) Necrotic tissue.

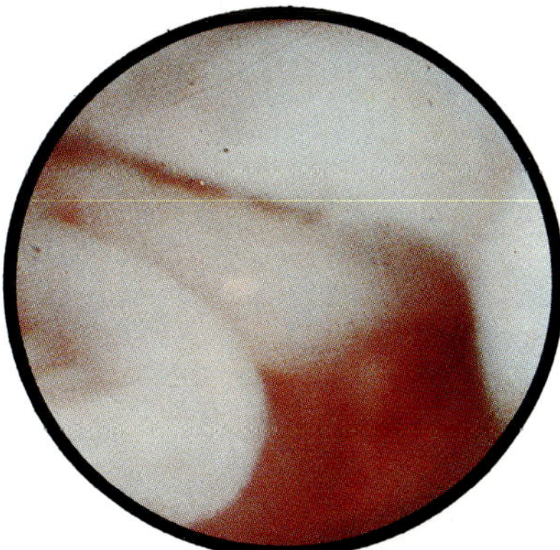

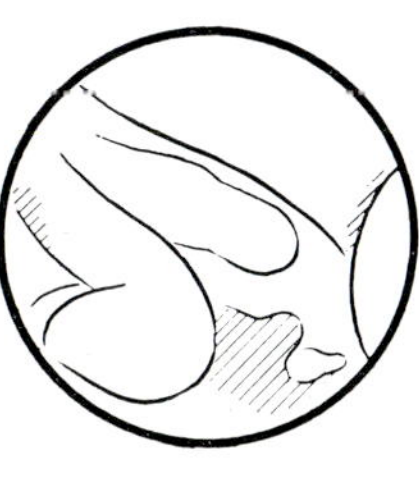

Fig. 121 A 50-year-old woman with rheumatoid arthritis of the right wrist joint, dorsoulnar approach. Swollen, opaque villi fill the joint cavity.

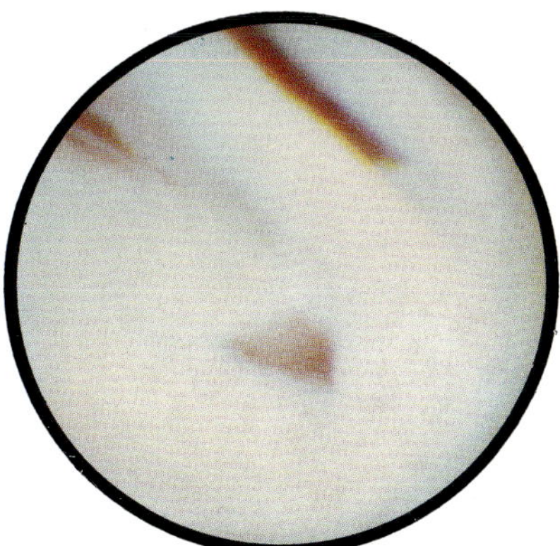

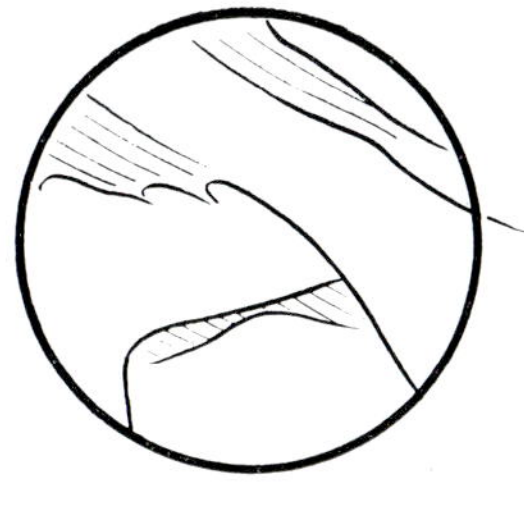

Fig. 122 Same patient as in Fig. 121. Cord-like necrotic tissue is seen.

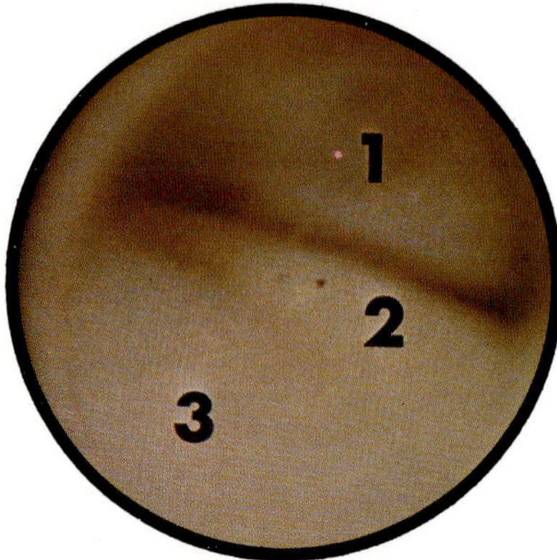

Fig. 123 A 31-year-old woman with rheumatoid arthritis of the left wrist, dorsoradial approach. (1) Radius. (2) Intercarpal ligament. (3) Scaphoid.

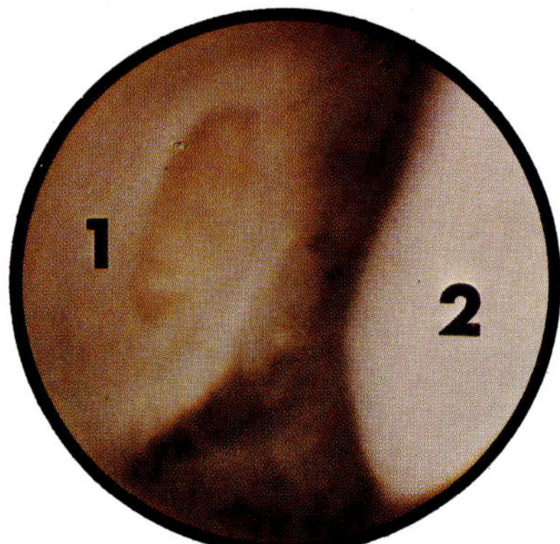

Fig. 124 A 39-year-old woman with rheumatoid arthritis of the right wrist, dorsoulnar approach. (1) Articular disk. (2) Os lunatum.

7

Arthroscopy of the Finger Joints

The No. 24 Watanabe arthroscope, developed in 1970, was the first instrument small enough to permit arthroscopy of the finger joints. Presented here are the results of arthroscopy of the finger joints performed on 28 amputated joints and 39 clinical cases (Tables 15 and 16).

ARTHROSCOPIC ANATOMY OF THE FINGER JOINTS

The Metacarpophalangeal Joint

The metacarpophalangeal joint (Fig. 125) is formed by the metacarpal head and the proximal end of the first phalanx. The metacarpophalangeal joint has one palmar and two collateral ligaments. Because it is a condyloid joint, it permits lateral deviation (abduction and adduction) in addition to flexion and extension. By traction on the metacarpophalangeal joint, two depressions can be palapated in the dorsal joint line alongside the extensor tendon. The depression palpated either radial or ulnar to the extensor tendon is a good landmark for guidance to the radial or ulnar dorsal approach.

Table 15 Clinical cases

Rheumatoid arthritis	29
Traumatic arthritis	2
Nonspecific synovitis	2
Fracture	2
Suppurative arthritis	1
Enchondroma	1
Extensor tendon rupture	1
Posttraumatic contracture	1
Total	39

Table 16 Arthroscopy of the finger joints

Joints examined	Clinical cases (joints)	Amputated joints
Metacarpophalangeal joint	31	10
Proximal interphalangeal joint	8	8
Distal interphalangeal joint	1	8
First interphalangeal joint	0	2
Totals	40	28

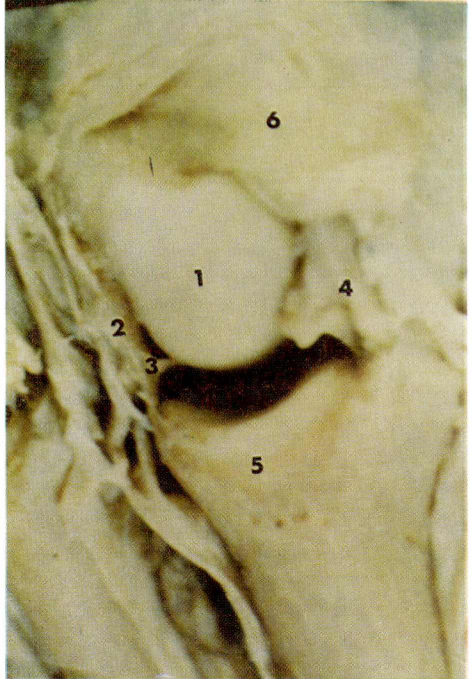

Fig. 125 Metacarpophalangeal joint of the right index finger. (1) Metacarpal head. (2) Ulnar collateral ligament. (3) Meniscus. (4) Radial collateral ligament. (5) Proximal phalanx. (6) Capsule.

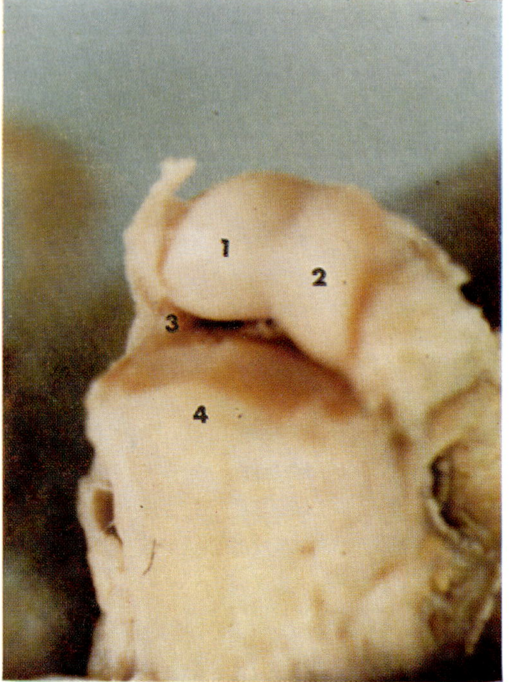

Fig. 126 Proximal interphalangeal joint. (1, 2) Condyles of proximal phalanx. (3) Ulnar collateral ligament. (4) Middle phalanx.

A proximal synovial recess—which can be divided into one dorsal and two lateral (radial and ulnar) recesses—is present in the metacarpophalangeal joint. The marginal meniscus projects into the interior of the joint, separating the peripheral part of the proximal articular surface of the first phalanx from direct contact with the metacarpal head.

The Interphalangeal Joints

The interphalangeal joints (interphalangeal joint of the thumb; proximal and distal interphalangeal joints) (Fig. 126) are hinge joints. Flexion and extension are their only movements. Each joint has one palmar and two collateral ligaments. The arrangement of these ligaments is similar to those in the metacarpophalangeal joint. The dorsal joint capsule usually has a plica and is difficult to separate from the extensor tendon.

TECHNIQUES (Fig. 127)

The instruments are sterilized by 24 hours' exposure in formalin gas chamber.

Finger joints) are easily anesthetized by local infiltration with 1% procaine or 1% lidocaine (Xylocaine). When finger joint examination is to be combined with an examination of other joints (shoulder, elbow, or wrist), brachial block, axillary block, or general anesthesia is recommended.

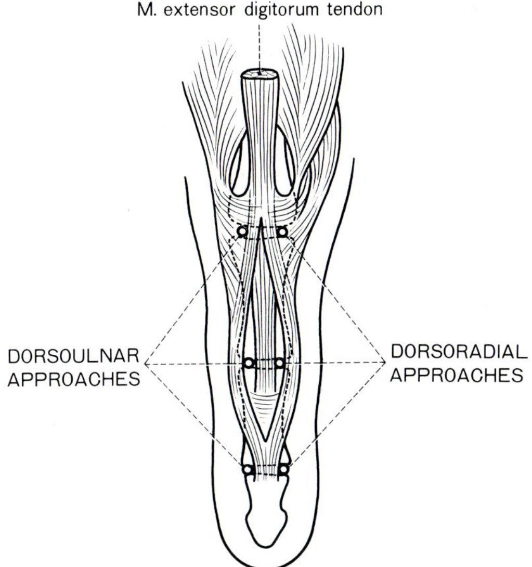

Fig. 127 Approaches of arthroscopy of the finger joints.

APPROACHES

Arthroscopy of the finger joints is carried out through dorsal approaches. The dorsal joint line is carefully determined, and traction is applied in mild flexion of the joint. The trocar puncture is made at the dorsal joint line—either radial (dorsoradial approach) or ulnar (dorsoulnar approach)—to the extensor tendon of the finger. The trocar is inserted obliquely into the dorsal joint cavity.

Traction on the finger during observation is effective in widening the visual field. Care should be taken that the tip of the arthroscope does not slip out of the joint during examination, as the finger joint cavities are very narrow. It is imperative that an assistant continuously inject normal saline solution into the joint to keep the joint cavity sufficiently distended and to obtain a clear visual field.

By either the dorsoradial or the dorsoulnar approach in the finger joints, the dorsal joint capsule, the joint space, the articular surfaces, the collateral ligaments, and the meniscus of the metacarpophalangeal joint can be observed. Examples are shown in Figures 128 through 137.

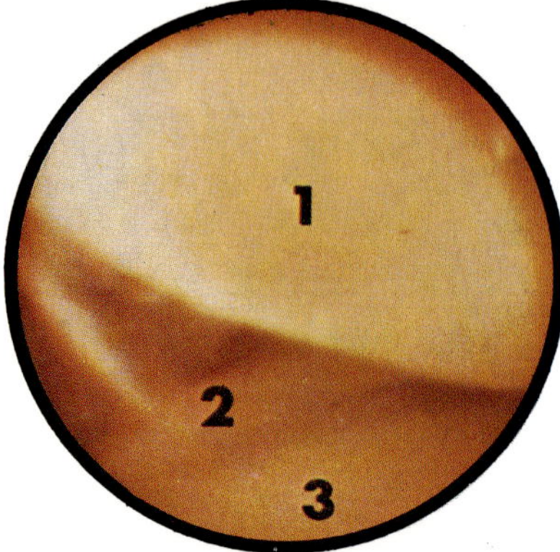

Fig. 128 Left fifth metacarpophalangeal joint of an amputation case, dorsoulnar approach. (1) Metacarpal head. (2) Meniscus. (3) Proximal phalanx.

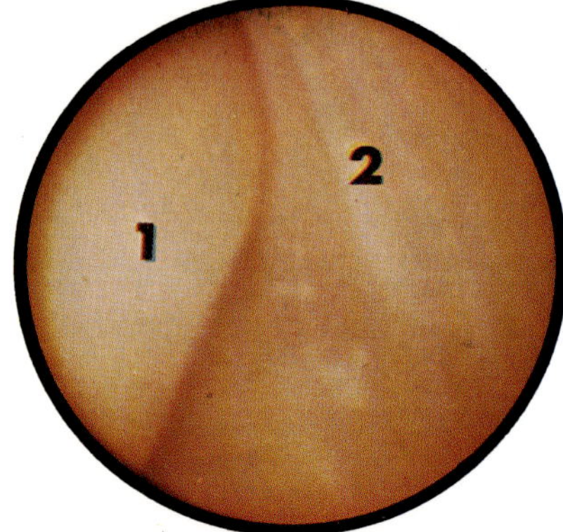

Fig. 129 Left third metacarpophalangeal joint of an amputation case, dorsoulnar approach. (1) Metacarpal head. (2) Ulnar collateral ligament.

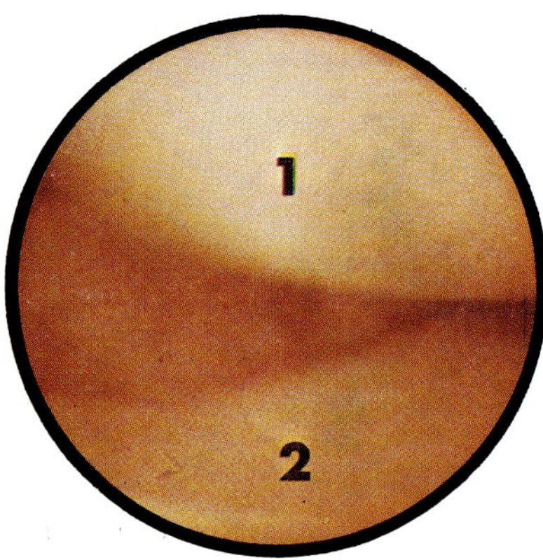

Fig. 130 Interphalangeal joint of the left thumb of an amputation case, dorsoulnar approach. (1) Condyle of the proximal phalanx. (2) Distal phalanx.

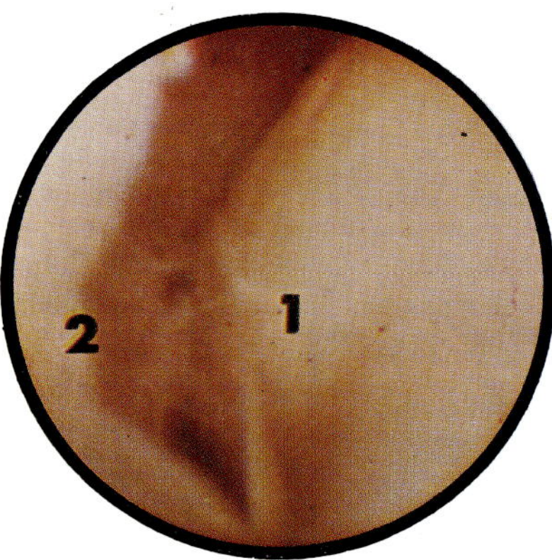

Fig. 131 Interphalangeal joint of the right thumb of an amputation case, dorsoradial approach. (1) Condyle of the proximal phalanx. (2) Dorsal wall.

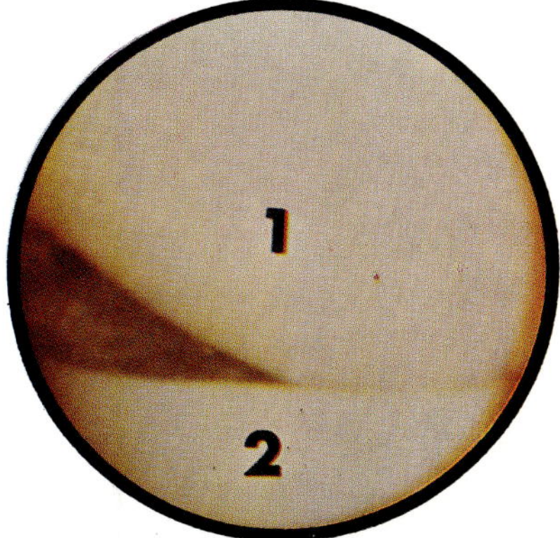

Fig. 132 Proximal interphalangeal joint of the left index finger of an amputation case, dorsoulnar approach. (1) (1) Proximal phalanx. (2) Middle phalanx.

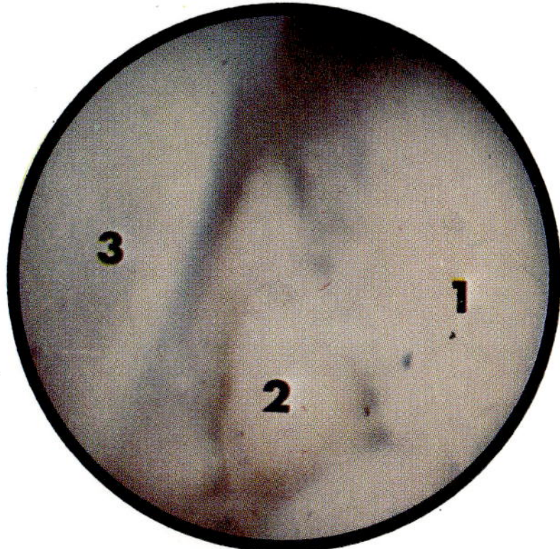

Fig. 133 A 51-year-old woman with rheumatoid arthritis of the metacarpophalangeal joint of the right thumb, dorsoradial approach. (1) Metacarpal head. (2) Villi. (3) Proximal phalanx.

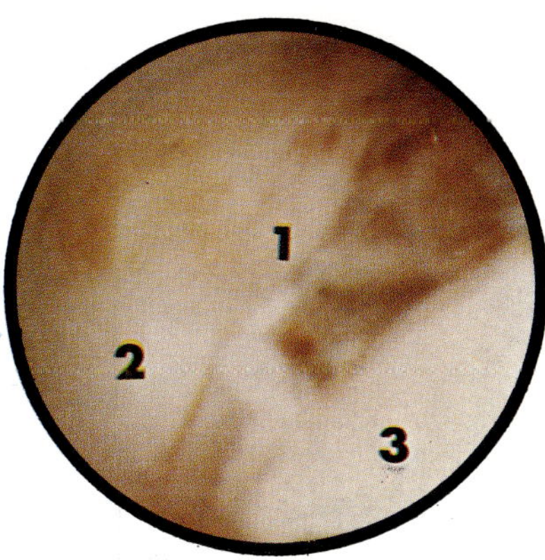

Fig. 134 A 45-year-old woman with rheumatoid arthritis of the metacarpophalangeal joint of the right middle finger, dorsoradial approach. (1) Necrotic and inflammatory villi. (2) Proximal phalanx. (3) Metacarpal head.

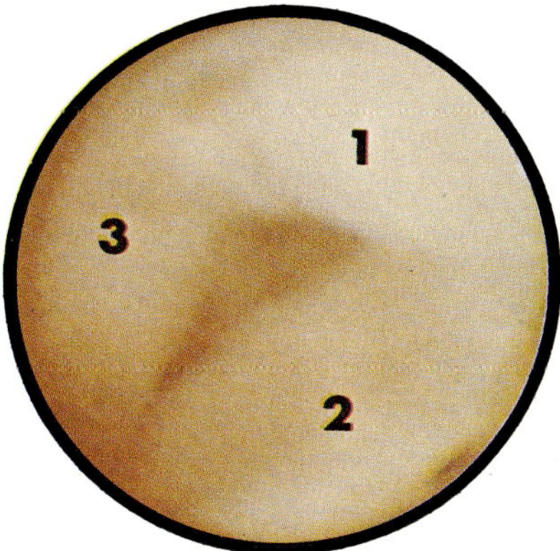

Fig. 135 A 28-year-old woman with rheumatoid arthritis of the proximal interphalangeal joint of the right middle finger, dorsoradial approach. (1) Villi. (2) Proximal phalanx. (3) Middle phalanx.

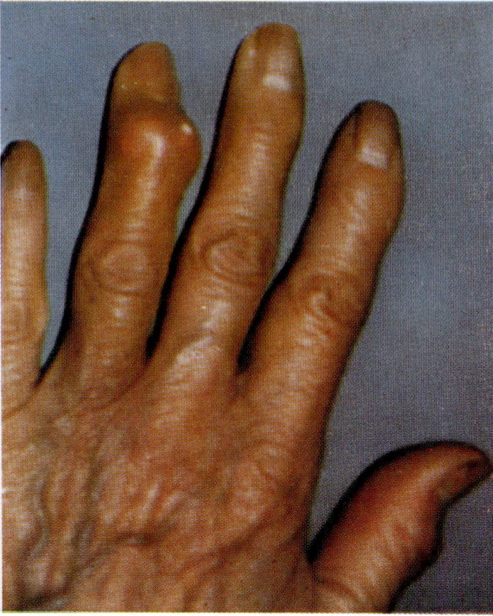

Fig. 136 An 80-year-old woman with gouty arthritis of the left hand.

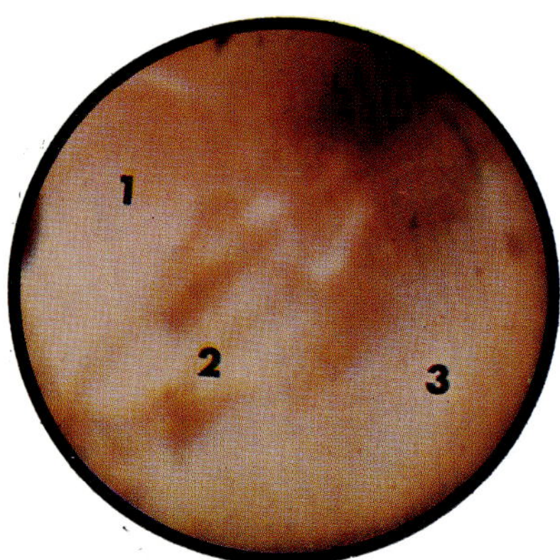

Fig. 137 An 80-year-old woman with gouty arthritis of the left fourth distal interphalangeal joint, dorsoulnar approach. (Same case as Fig. 136) (1) Distal phalanx. (2) Urate crystal. (3) Middle phalanx.

8

Arthroscopy of the Hip Joint

ANATOMY

The hip joint is a typical ball and socket joint, consisting of the femoral head and the acetabulum. The femoral head is ball-shaped and there is a fovea in the central portion in which the ligamentum teres is embedded. The central portion of the acetabulum also makes a deeply depressed fovea, which is the acetabular notch. The notch is covered with the transverse acetabular ligament and the synovial membrane. The glenoid limbus goes around the acetabulum (Fig. 138). The limbus of the articular cavity accounts for its large size, with the acetabulum covering more than half of the femoral head (Fig. 139). The articular surface of the acetabulum is restricted to the articular crescent (facies lunata) (Fig. 140). In the acetabulum, the ligamentum teres attaches to the notch. The ligamentum teres consists of three bundles. The posterior ischial bundle (the longest) runs through the

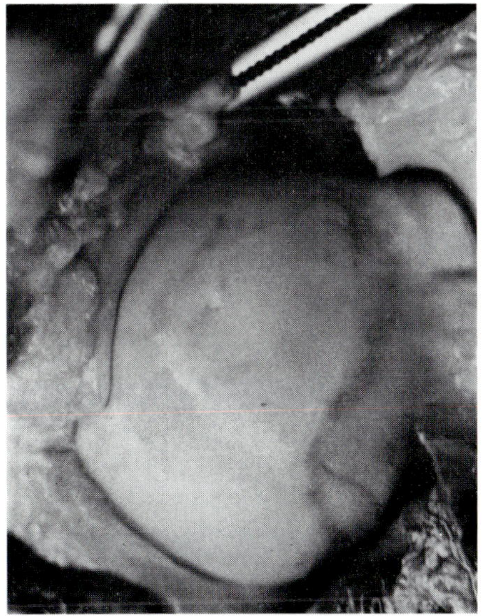

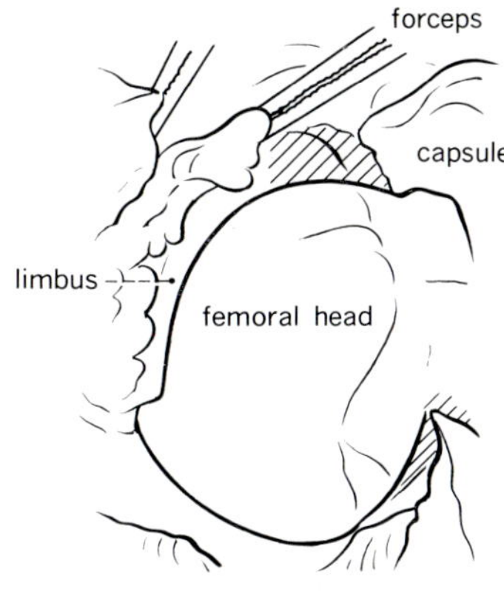

Fig. 138 The acetabular limbus and the femoral head.

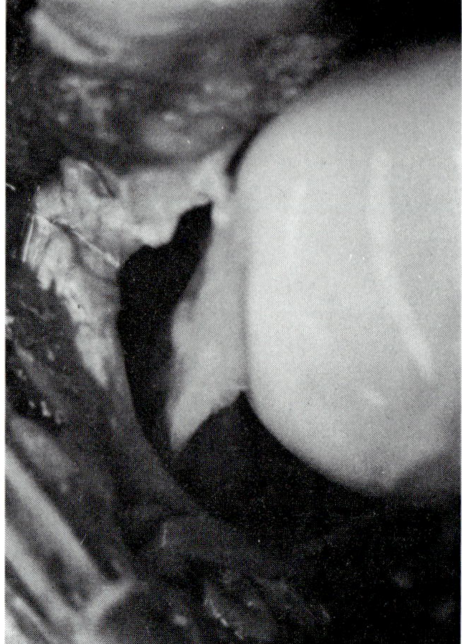

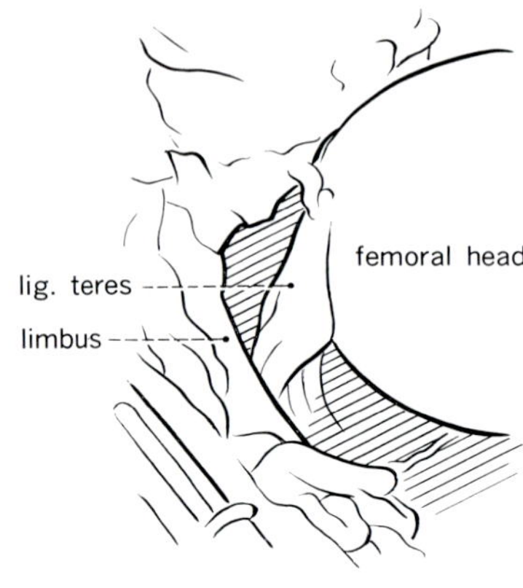

Fig. 139 The ligamentum teres, the femoral head, and the acetabulum.

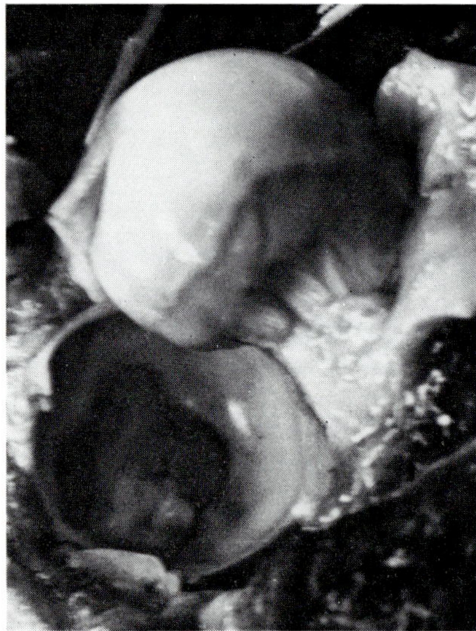

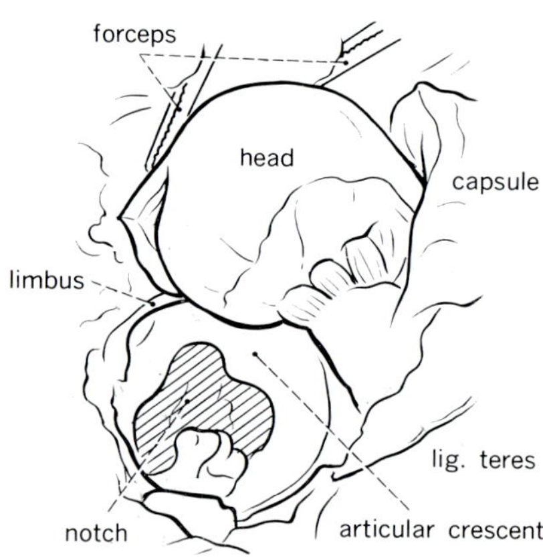

Fig. 140 The articular crescent and the notch in the acetabulum.

acetabular notch, under the transverse ligament, and inserts below and behind the posterior horn of the horseshoe-shaped acetabular crescent. The anterior pubic bundle inserts into the acetabular notch behind the anterior horn of the articular crescent. The intermediate bundle (the thinnest) is inserted into the upper border of the transverse ligament.

The capsule is very thick. It begins at the rim of the acetabulum and covers the femoral head. The anterior portion lies embedded in the linea intertrochanterica, and the posterior portion is embedded in the femoral neck. Supplement ligaments, include the ligamentum iliocapsulare, located posteriorly; the ligamentum pubocapsulare, located medially; and the ligamentum iliofemorale, located anteriorly.

CLINICAL EXPERIENCES

From 1974 to 1983, 47 arthroscopic studies of the hip joint were performed on 40 joints in 37 patients (12 male, 25 female) (Table 17). Twenty-five right hips, fifteen left hips, and three bilateral cases were examined. The patents' ages ranged from 4 months to 60 years, with a mean age of 30 years. General anesthesia was used seven times, lumbar anesthesia six times, continuous epidural anesthesia 30 times, and local anesthesia four times.

PROCEDURE

The anterolateral approach (Fig. 141) was employed in all cases. Basically, the insertion place was the point at which the saggital line through the anterior iliac spine crossed with the horizontal line through the proximal top of the major trochanter. The angle of direction was pointed toward the hip joint line.

The anterolateral approach is not difficult in children, but is difficult in adults, especially in cases of osteoarthritis. For osteoarthritic cases, it is helpful to raise the patient's buttocks

Table 17 Arthroscopy of the hip joint

Condition	Number of patients	Number of joints	Number of times
Pain in a joint	1	1	1
Contracture after fractures	2	2	2
Congenitally dislocated hip	8	9	11
Perthes' disease	4	4	5
Slipped capital epiphysis	1	1	1
Aseptic necrosis	2	2	2
Osteoarthritis	14	16	19
Rheumatoid arthritis	4	4	5
Coxitis	1	1	1
Total	37	40	47

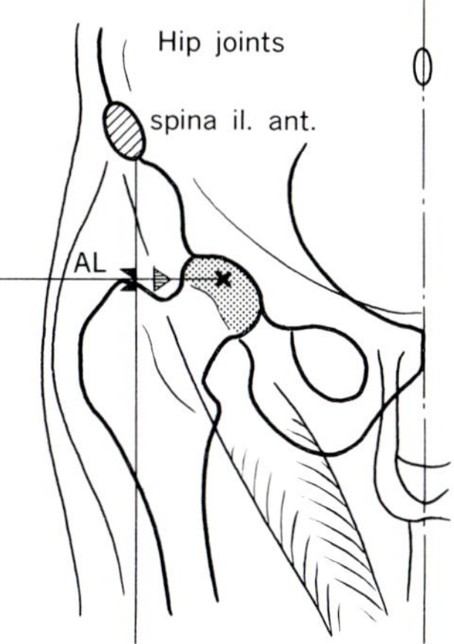

Fig. 141 Anterolateral approach to the right hip.

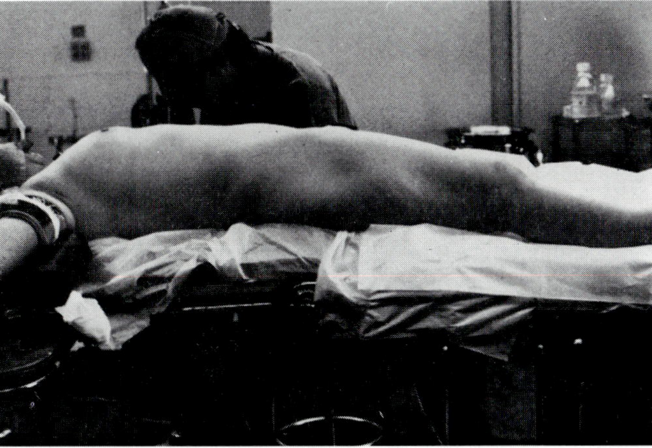

Fig. 142 Position for the hip arthroscopy.

with a hard pillow and to keep the hip in a slight hyperextended position (Fig. 142). When the tip of the needle reaches the capsule the hip joint is slightly flexed and the needle can be introduced to the joint cavity.

The visible field of the acetabulum (Fig. 143) is very narrow, but, through manipulation, the field widens in the femoral head.

CLINICAL CASES

Case 1 A 7-year-old boy with Perthes' disease on the right (Fig. 144).
Two months before presentation, claudication occurred. On August 25, 1978, arthroscopy was performed. The articular cartilage had lost its gloss and was uneven. The acetabulum was observed with the limbus, and the ligamentum teres was partially seen. The distal anteromedial portion of the joint cavity was also well observed.

Case 2 A 9-year-old girl with Perthes' disease on the left (Fig. 145).
Arthroscopy was performed on March 16, 1977. The medial surface of the femoral head was remarkably uneven and a part of it was depressed. The cartilage of the acetabulum had lost its gloss and the color was brownish. Except for the posterior

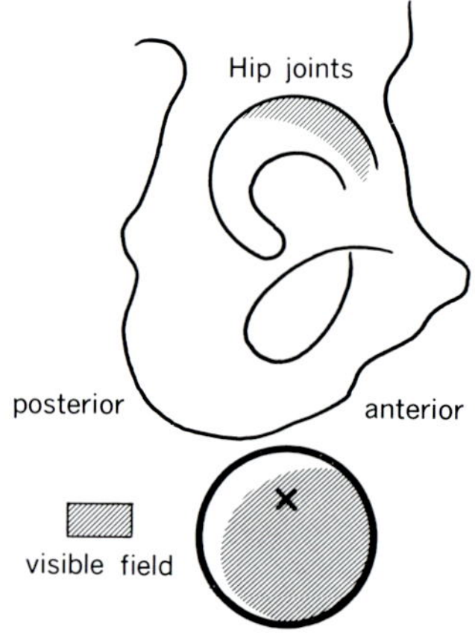

Fig. 143 Visible field of the hip.

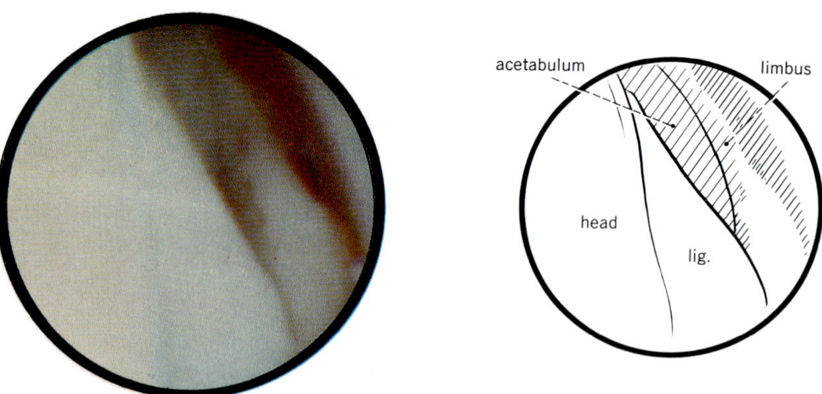

Fig. 144 The ligamentum teres, the femoral head, the limbus, and the acetabulum.

portion of the acetabulum and the joint cavity, almost the whole surface of the articular cartilage with the limbus was well observed because of easy manipulation of the joint.

Case 3 A 14-year-old boy with slipped capital epiphysis of the right femur (Figs. 146 and 147). In July 1975, while playing baseball, the patient had pain in the right hip. The hip was treated conservatively. Arthroscopy on February 8, 1978 resulted in a diagnosis of coxa adolescentia. The acetabulum revealed fibrous changes (Fig. 146) with a proliferation of hyperemic villi in the joint cavity (Fig. 147). On February 24, 1978, osteotomy was carried out.

Case 4 A 43-year-old woman with secondary osteoarthritis of the right hip (Fig. 148). In 1970, at the age of 32 years, the patient presented with a complaint of pain in the hip. Arthroscopy performed on March 3, 1972, revealed fibrillation changes on the femoral head. In 1981, pain in the hip recurred. On August 3, 1981, a roentgenogram was taken and on August 7, 1981, a shelf operation was carried out following arthroscopic examination. The arthroscopic examination had revealed step-wise changes from the anterior to the posterior in the boundary between the non-weight-bearing portion and the weight-bearing portion on the articular surface of the femoral head. In the non-weight-bearing portion, which is the dislocated lateral portion of the head, the articular cartilage was in the process of disappearing. In the lateral edge of the remaining articular cartilage, the cartilage seemed to be breaking off. In the anterior portion of the head, a small ulcer surrounded with fibrillation changes was found. The limbus was

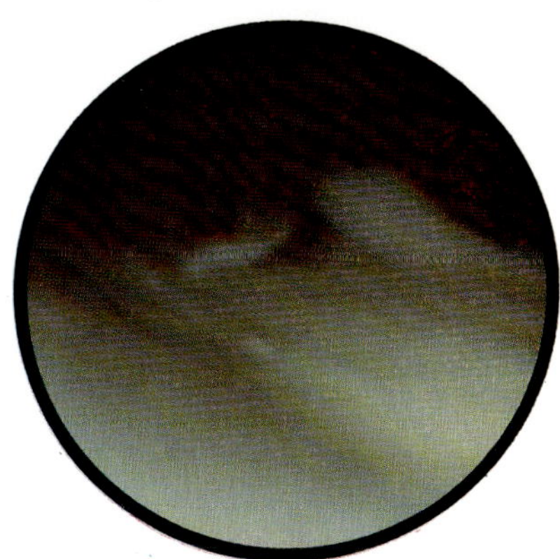

Fig. 145 Rough surfaces of the femoral head.

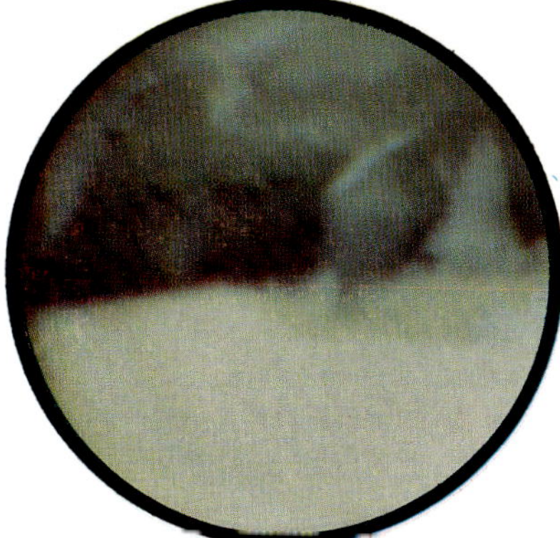

Fig. 146 Fibrillation changes in the acetabulum.

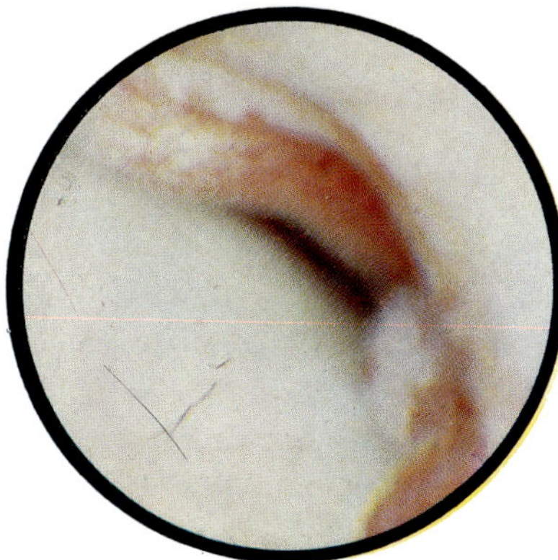

Fig. 147 Hyperemic villi in the left hip.

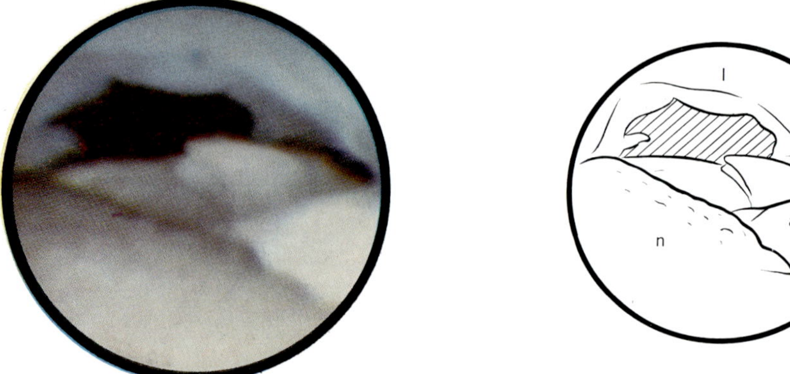

Fig. 148 Step-wise changes of the articular cartilage of the femoral head. The left side is the non-weight-bearing area in which the articular cartilage was in the process of disappearing. (n) Non-weight-bearing area. (a) Articular cartilage. (l) Limbus.

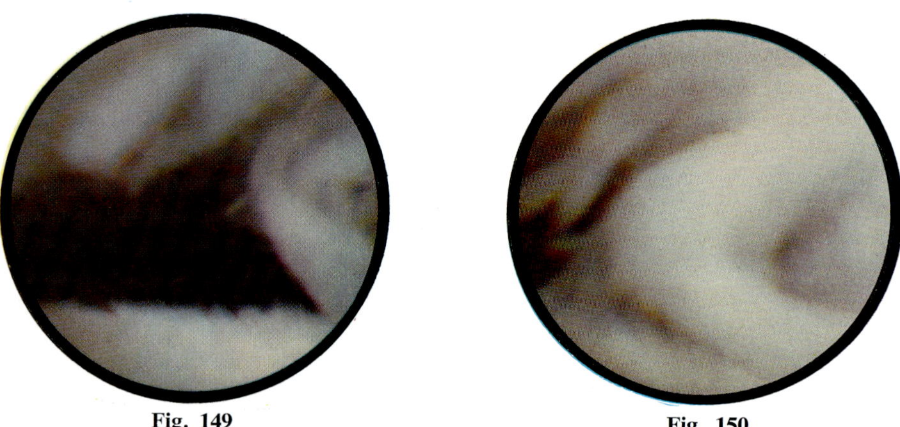

Fig. 149 **Fig. 150**

Figs. 149, 150 Fibrous changes and necrotic tissues.

observed and the acetabulum showed fibrous changes with a proliferation of fibrous villi in the front synovium. The patient has no complaints at present.

Case 5 A 52-year-old woman with secondary osteoarthritis of the right hip (Figs. 149 and 150).

On August 5, 1980, arthroscopy was performed. Fibrous tissues filled the joint cavity. The articular cartilage of the femoral head had mostly disintegrated. The acetabulum revealed fibrillation changes. On the same day, debridement of the joint with a shelf operation was carried out. At present the patient has no complaints of pain, and her walking distances are unrestricted.

Case 6 A 47-year-old woman with nonspecific chronic coxitis on the right (Fig. 151).

In December 1961, pain in the left hip joint occurred. It was treated conservatively. On September 10, 1975, arthroscopy was performed, revealing that the femoral head had lost its gloss and was uneven. There were necrotic masses and granulation tissues in the joint cavity. The inflammatory condition seemed to have subsided. The patient had no complaints of pain or limitation of motion in the right hip in February 1980.

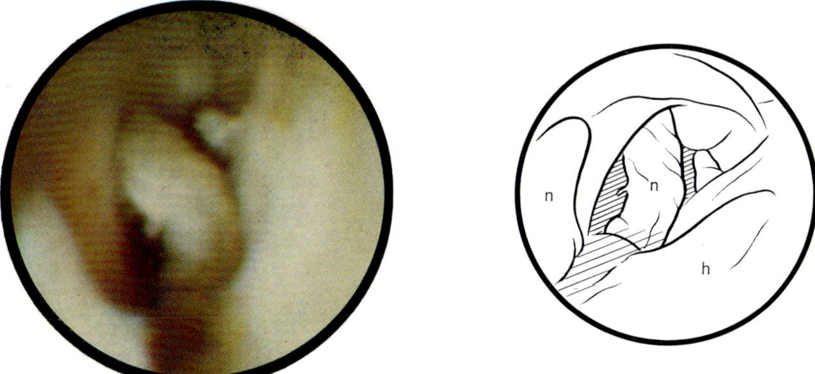

Fig. 151 Rough surfaces of the femoral head with necrotic masses. (h) Rough surface of the femoral head. (n) Fibrous tissues and necrotic masses.

9

Arthroscopy of the Ankle Joint

ARTHROSCOPIC ANATOMY OF THE ANKLE JOINT

The ankle joint is composed of the lower end of the tibia with its medial malleolus and lateral malleolus, as well as the trochlea, medial, and lateral malleolar surfaces of the talus. The ankle joint (Fig. 152) can be subdivided into four joints—the distal tibiofibular joint, the middle (or proper) talocrural joint, and the medial and lateral talocrural (or talomalleolar) joints—and six pouches—the anterior, anteromedial, anterolateral, posterior, posteromedial, and posterolateral pouches.

The capsular ligament is attached proximally to the margins of the tibial and fibular epiphyses and distally to the margin of the superior articular surface of the talus except anteriorly, where it extends forward to the neck of the talus. The capsular ligament is relatively fragile, especially anteriorly and posteriorly, and forms prominent pouches that allow plantar flexion and dorsiflexion of the ankle joint.

The deltoid ligament (Fig. 153) strengthens the medial side of the joint with a deep band running from the medial malleolus to the talus and a superficial layer that is divided into three bands, i.e., the tibionavicular, tibiocalcaneal, and posterior tibiotalar ligaments. Laterally, three distinct ligaments (Fig. 154) are present, i.e., the anterior talofibular, the

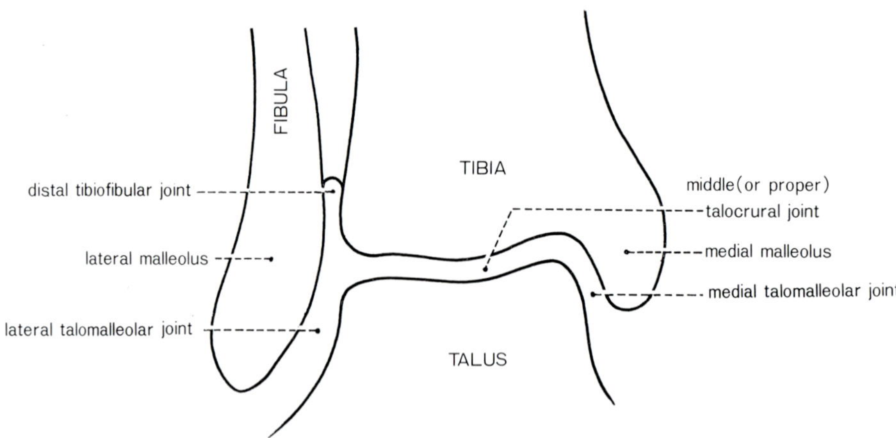

Fig. 152 Subdivision of the talocrural joint.

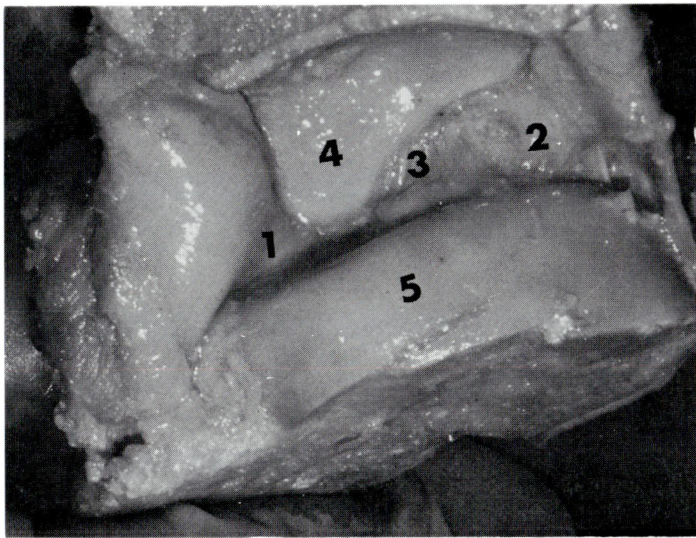

Fig. 153 Medial compartment of the left ankle joint. (1) Anteromedial pouch. (2) Posteromedial pouch. (3) Deltoid ligament. (4) Medial malleolus. (5) Talus.

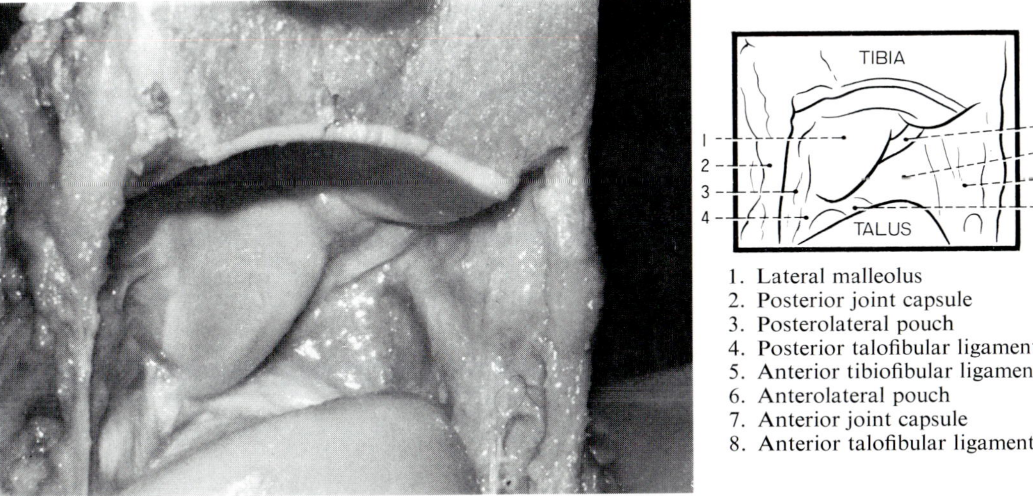

Fig. 154 Lateral compartment of the left ankle joint.

calcaneofibular, and the posterior talofibular ligaments. The posterior talofibular ligament usually extends a tibial slip attaching to the posterior tibia.

The tibia and fibula of the distal tibiofibular joint are connected by the strong interosseous ligament and the anterior and posterior tibiofibular ligaments. The distal tibiofibular joint moves laterally about 1 mm to 3 mm in dorsiflexion of the ankle joint. This is because the superior surface of the talus is wider in front than behind. Hence, the ankle mortise is wider in dorsiflexion of the joint, and lateral movements at the ankle mortise occur more freely in plantar flexion than dorsiflexion of the joint.

The synovial membrane covers the capsular ligament, the deltoid ligament, the anterior and posterior talofibular ligaments, and the recess of the distal tibiofibular joint.

The joint space of the proper talocrural joint (Fig. 155) is convex in the anteroposterior direction and concave from side to side (Fig. 156). The medial talomalleolar joint space (Fig. 157) is flat and oblique medially. The lateral talomalleolar joint space (Fig. 158) is more oblique as compared with the medial talomalleolar joint space, and is concave laterally near the tip of the lateral malleolus. The distal tibiofibular joint is an apposition of the convex fibular surface and the concave tibial surface, and permits some lateral movement in dorsiflexion of the ankle joint. There is a tibiofibular joint cavity of 5 mm to 12 mm (average, 6.5 mm) in depth, with a lining of synovial membrane. The opening of the distal tibiofibular joint is always covered by a cartilaginous plica (Fig. 159).

Fat pads (Figs. 160, 161) of various sizes and shapes are usually seen at the four corners (anteromedial, anterolateral, posteromedial, and posterolateral) of the ankle joint. The

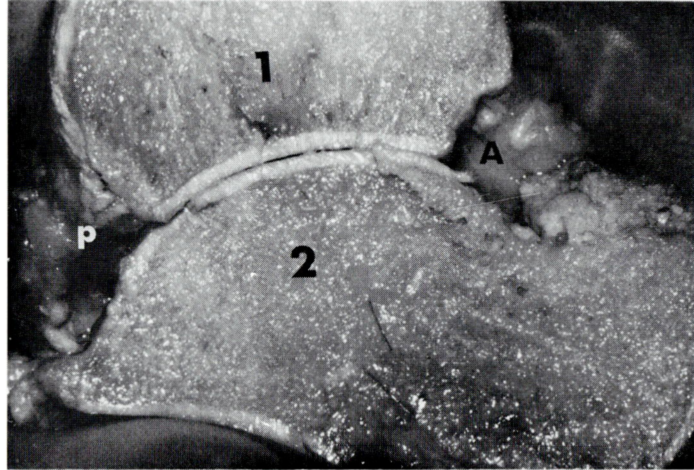

Fig. 155 Sagittal section of the left ankle joint. (A) Anterior pouch. (P) Posterior pouch. (1) Tibia. (2) Talus.

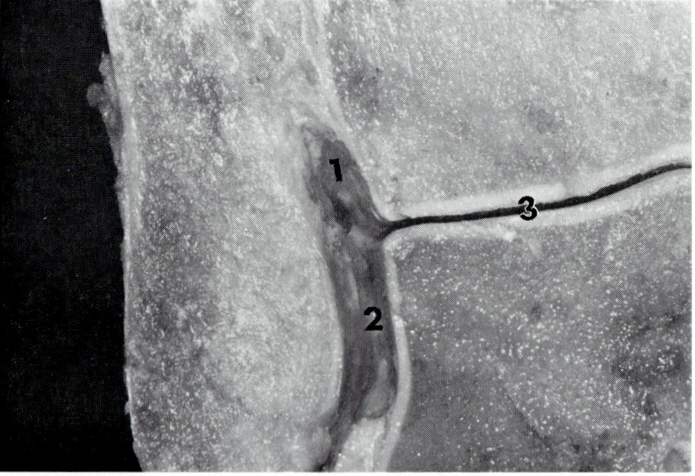

Fig. 156 Frontal section of the right ankle joint. (1) Distal tibiofibular joint. (2) Lateral talomalleolar joint. (3) Middle talocrural joint.

surface of the fat pad is smooth to granularly coarse, and it may be lobulated. These fat pads may interfere with the observation of the joint.

The anterior margin of the lower tibia is slightly convex in anterodistal direction. There is a medial notch (Fig. 162) of the lower tibia near the anterior junction of the medial malleolus. Hence, the anteromedial approach may permit a better view for examining the whole joint space of the proper talocrural joint. The tip of the arthroscope can also reach the posterior pouch through the anteromedial approach.

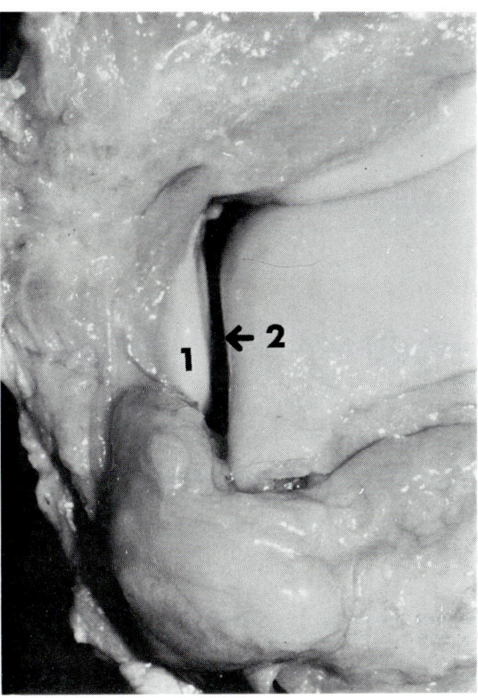

Fig. 157 Medial talomalleolar joint (left ankle) (1) Medial malleolus. (2) Medial talomalleolar joint.

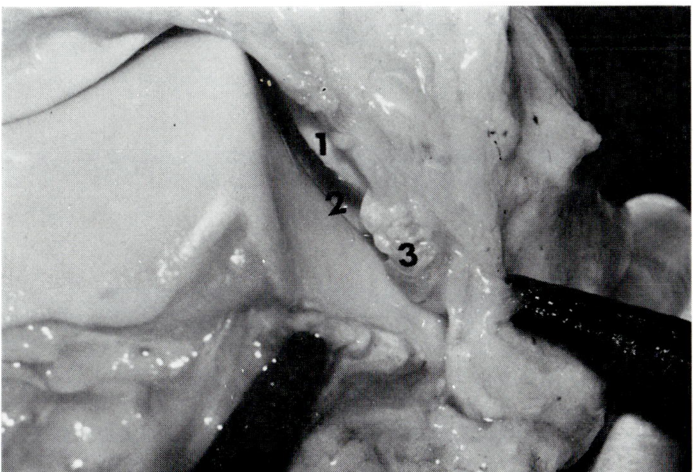

Fig. 158 Lateral talomalleolar (or talofibular) joint (left ankle). (1) Lateral malleolus. (2) Talofibular joint. (3) Anterior talofibular ligament.

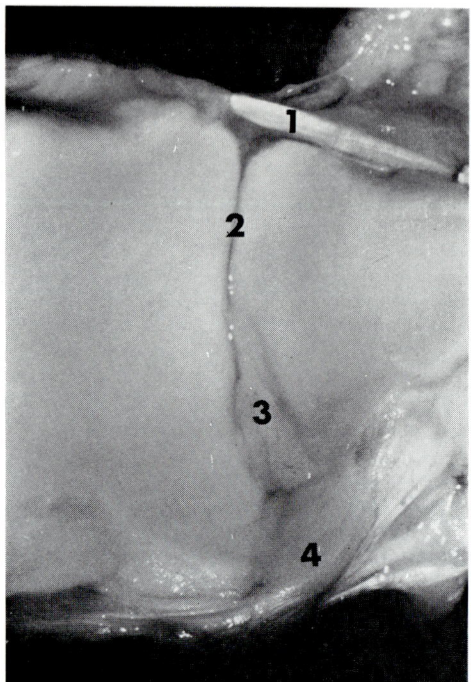

Fig. 159 Distal tibiofibular joint. (1) Anterior tibiofibular ligament. (2) Distal tibiofibular joint. (3) Cartilaginous plica. (4) Posterior tibiofibular ligament.

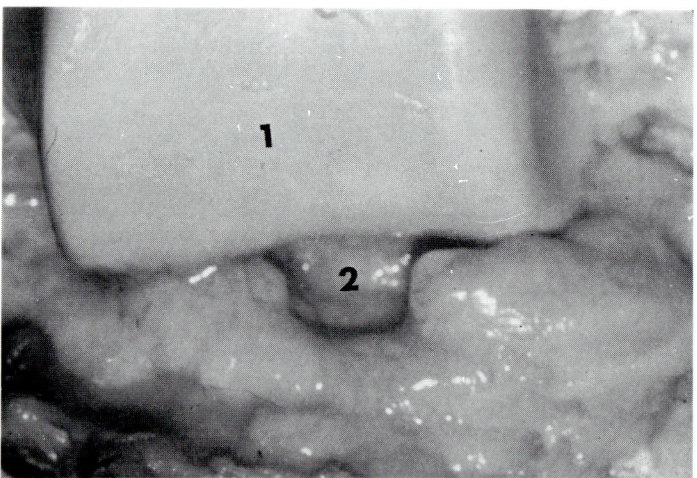

Fig. 160 Anterior compartment of the right ankle joint. (1) Talus. (2) Anterior recess.

NORMAL ARTHROSCOPIC VIEWS OF THE ANKLE JOINT

The arthroscopic views observed in the normal ankle joint are sketched in Figure 163.

1. Anterior pouch—anterior recess, anterior synovial wall, fat pads, anterior tibiofibular ligament
2. Anteromedial pouch—medial synovial wall, medial malleolus, medial malleolar surface of the talus, deltoid ligament

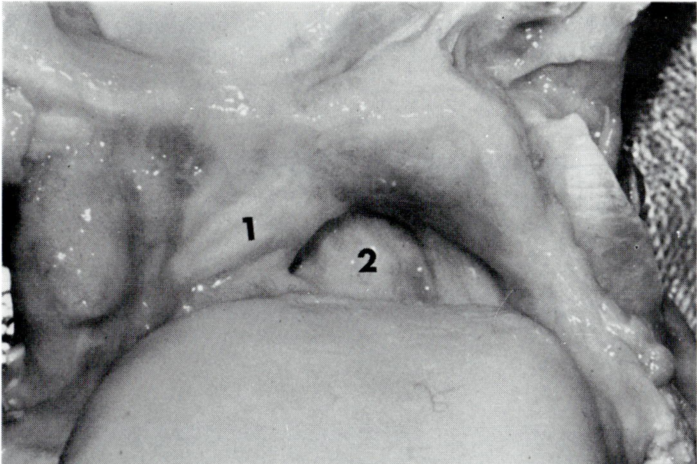

Fig. 161 Posterior compartment of the right ankle joint. (1) Tibial slip of the posterior talofibular ligament. (2) Posterior recess.

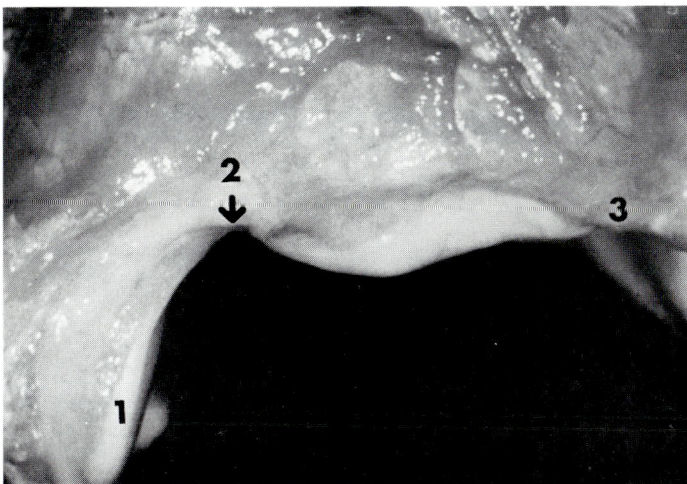

Fig. 162 Anterior view of the proximal part of the left ankle joint. (1) Medial malleolus. (2) Notch. (3) Anterior tibiofibular ligament.

3. Anterolateral pouch—lateral synovial wall, lateral malleolus, lateral malleolar surface of the talus, anterior talofibular ligament
4. Posterior pouch—posterior recess, fat pad, posterior tibiofibular ligament, tibial slip of the posterior talofibular ligament
5. Posteromedial pouch—medial synovial wall, deltoid ligament
6. Posterolateral pouch—lateral synovial wall, lateral malleolus, lateral malleolar surface of the talus, posterior talofibular ligament
7. Proper (or middle) talocrural joint—articular surface of the distal tibia, proximal talus
8. Medial talomalleolar joint—articular surface of the medial malleolus, medial articular surface of the talus, deltoid ligament

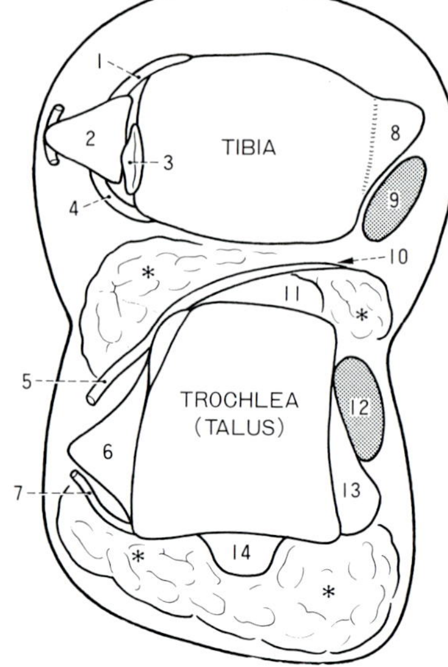

Fig. 163 Structures for arthroscopy (right ankle). (1) Anterior tibiofibular ligament. (2) Lateral malleolus. (3) Cartilaginous plica. (4) Posterior tibiofibular ligament. (5) Posterior talofibular ligament. (6) Lateral malleolar surface (talus). (7) Anterior talofibular ligament. (8) Medial malleolus. (9) Deltoid ligament. (10) Tibial slip of the posterior talofibular ligament. (11) Posterior recessus. (12) Deltoid ligament. (13) Medial malleolar surface (talus). (14) Anterior recessus.

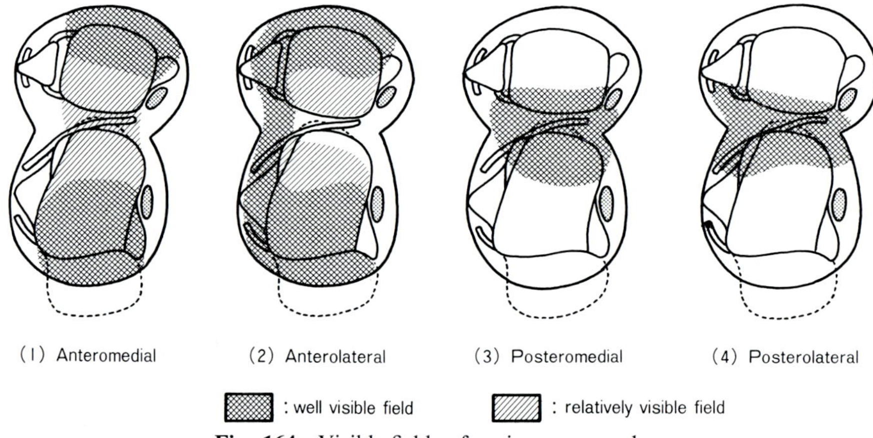

Fig. 164 Visible fields of various approaches.

9. Lateral talomalleolar (or talofibular) joint—articular surface of the lateral malleolus, lateral articular surface of the talus
10. Distal tibiofibular joint—orifice of the distal tibiofibular joint with its cartilaginous plica

All these parts of the ankle joint can not be examined by a single puncture. There are certain dead spaces beyond the arthroscopic view of each approach because of the anatomic complexity of the talocrural joint. For instance, the lateral compartment of the ankle joint and a part of the posterior pouch are dead space in the anteromedial approach. The dead space can be reduced by combined approaches, well-relaxing anesthesia, and improvement in operator technique gained through experience. The visible field of each approach is sketched in Figure 164. The selection of approaches for ankle joint arthroscopy is shown in Table 18.

The anterior pouch (Fig. 165) is the largest pouch of the ankle joint. The synovial wall

Table 18 Selection of approaches for ankle joint arthroscopy

Compartment	Approach			
	Anteromedial	Anterolateral	Posteromedial	Posterolateral
Anterior pouch	+	+	−	−
Anteromedial pouch	+	−	−	−
Anterolateral pouch	−	+	−	−
Posterior pouch	+	+	+	+
Posteromedial pouch	+	−	+	+
Posterolateral pouch	−	+	−	+
Proper talocrural joint	+	+	+	+
Medial talomalleolar joint	+	−	+	−
Lateral talomalleolar joint	−	+	−	+
Distal tibiofibular joint	+	+	+	+
Deltoid ligament	+	−	+	−
Anterior talofibular ligament	−	+	−	−
Posterior talofibular ligament	−	+	−	+
Anterior tibiofibular ligament	+	+	−	−
Posterior tibiofibular ligament	+	+	+	+
Tibial slip of the posterior talofibular ligament	+	+	+	+

+ = Visible. − = Not visible.

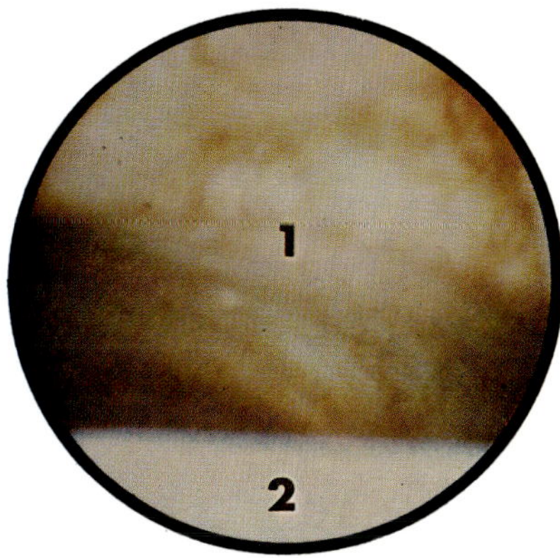

Fig. 165 Anterior pouch of the left ankle joint with anterolateral approach. (1) Anterior wall. (2) Talus.

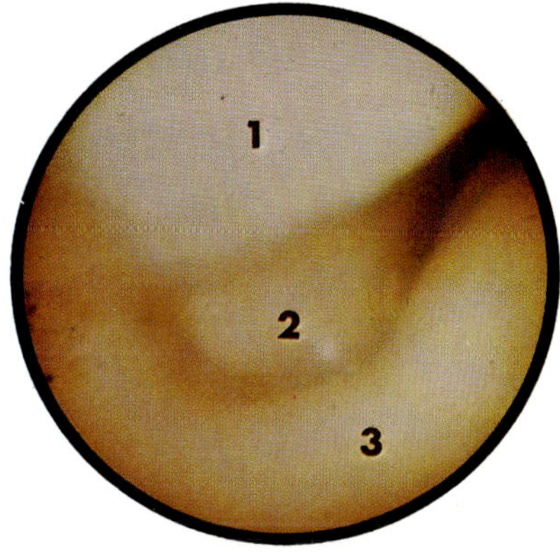

Fig. 166 Anterior pouch of the right ankle joint with anteromedial approach. (1) Talus. (2) Anterior recess. (3) Fat pad.

of the anterior pouch usually has few villi. The blood vessels on the surfaces of the synovial membrane and villi are clearly visible. Occasionally, the longitudinal band and/or the transverse fold of the synovial membrane can be seen on the anterior capsular wall. Transmission of pulsation from the dorsal pedis artery is often observed. There is a shallow anterior recess (Fig. 166) at the center, over the neck of the talus. On the sides of the anterior recess are two separated fat pads, or one fat pad thicker in both sides, extending to the anteromedial and anterolateral pouches. The transition of the anterior articular cartilage of the talus usually has a small gap.

As seen when the arthroscope is moved into the anteromedial pouch (Fig. 167), the medial malleolar tip is round, the medial malleolar surface of the talus is smooth, and the medial synovial wall often presents a striated appearance.

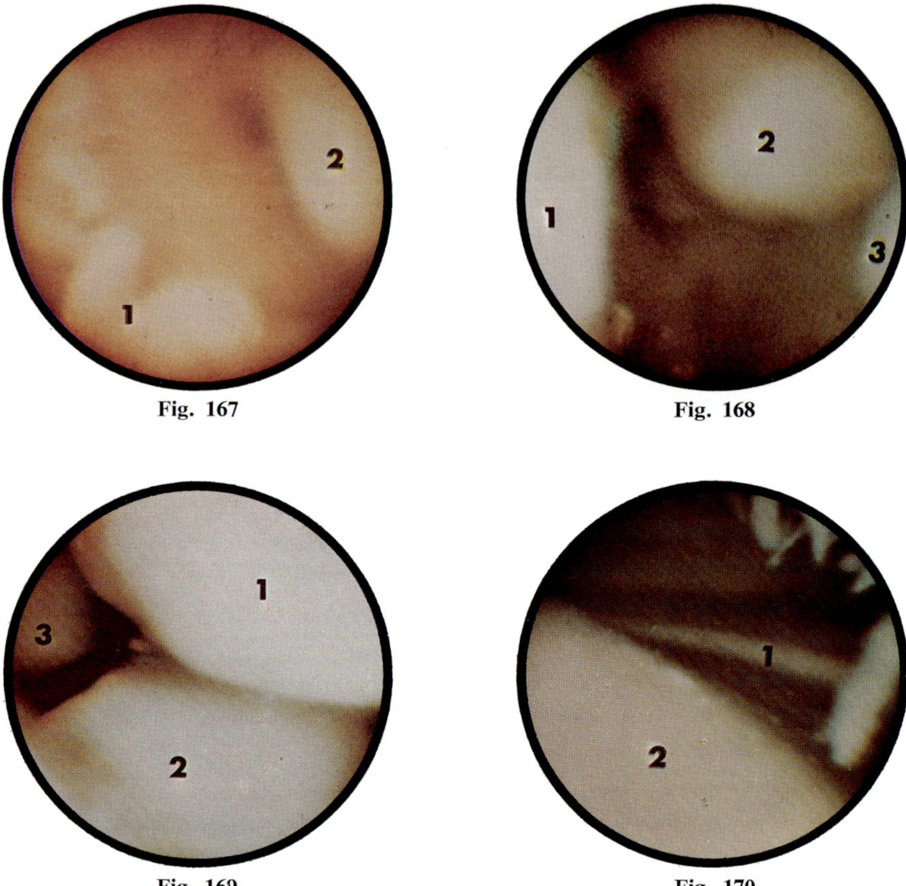

Fig. 167

Fig. 168

Fig. 169

Fig. 170

Fig. 167 Anteromedial pouch of the left ankle joint with anteromedial approach. (1) Villi. (2) Medial malleolus.

Fig. 168 Anterolateral pouch of the left ankle joint with anterolateral approach. (1) Talus. (2) Lateral malleolus. (3) Anterior talofibular ligament.

Fig. 169 Posterior pouch and posteromedial pouch of the right ankle joint with posterolateral approach. (1) Tibia. (2) Talus. (3) Fat pad in the posteromedial pouch.

Fig. 170 Tibial slip of the posterior talofibular ligament with anteromedial approach. (1) Tibial slip. (2) Talus.

On inspecting the anterolateral pouch (Fig. 168), one finds the space of the anterolateral pouch to be larger than the anteromedial pouch. The anterior talofibular ligament is identified between the lateral malleolar tip and the talus and it is tensed on plantar flexion with varus stress of the ankle joint, and relaxed on dorsiflexion of the ankle joint. The tip of the lateral malleolus also has a round appearance. Occasionally, longitudinal synovial pleats can be found on the lateral synovial wall. The lateral malleolar surface of the talus is deeper than the medial malleolar surface of the talus and it is concave laterally on frontal view.

Both capacities of the anteromedial and anterolateral pouches are diminished by dorsiflexion and enlarged by plantar flexion of the ankle joint.

The posterior pouch (Fig. 169), the second largest pouch of the ankle joint, usually has

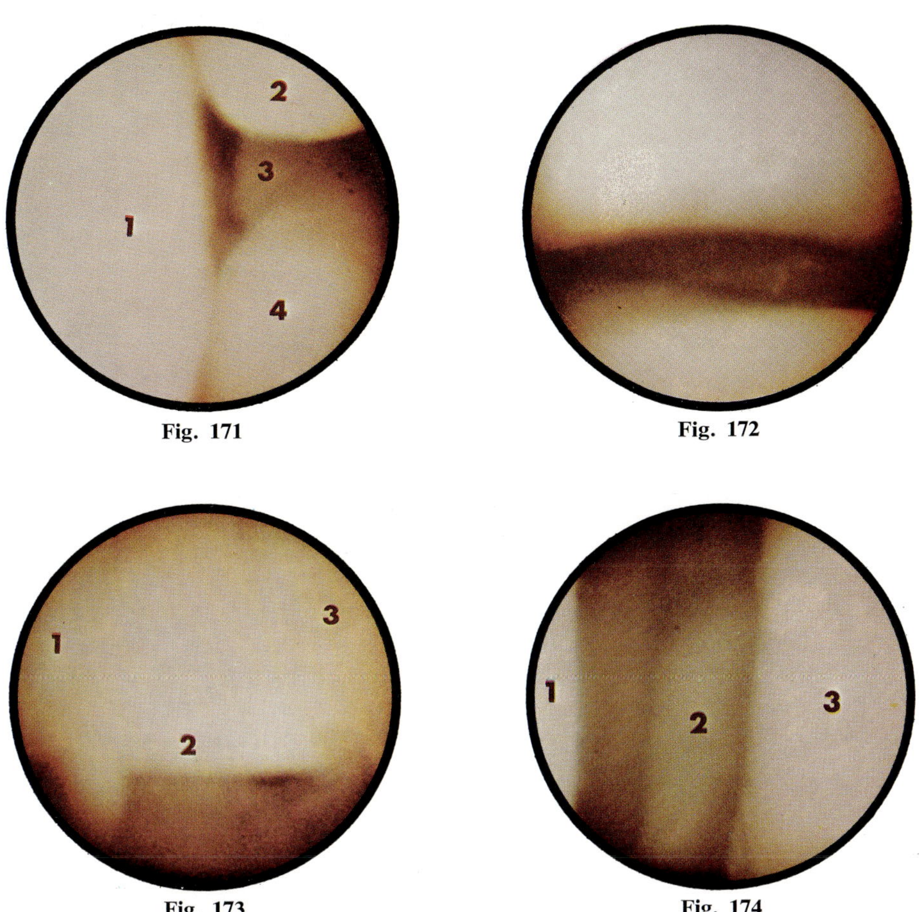

Fig. 171 Fig. 172

Fig. 173 Fig. 174

Fig. 171 Posterolateral pouch of the right ankle joint with posterolateral approach. (1) Talus. (2) Lateral malleolus. (3) Posterior talofibular ligament. (4) Fat pad in the posterolateral pouch.
Fig. 172 Middle (proper) talocrural joint (right ankle joint) with anteromedial approach.
Fig. 173 Medial talomalleolar joint of the left ankle with anteromedial approach. (1) Medial malleolus. (2) Deltoid ligament. (3) Talus.
Fig. 174 Lateral talomalleolar (talofibular) joint of the left ankle with anterolateral approach. (1) Talus. (2) Posterior talofibular ligament. (3) Lateral malleolus.

a small posterior recess located at the bottom of the posterior pouch, with or without a small valve at its opening. This posterior recess is seldom observed because of the obstruction of the fat pad at its opening. The tibial slip (Fig. 170) of the posterior talofibular ligament with its synovial membrane forms a transverse fold in the posterior pouch. It is best examined by posterior approaches, but can also be observed by the anteromedial approach.

The posteromedial pouch is very shallow and is the smallest pouch in the ankle joint. It often has a small fat pad on the medial synovial wall.

The posterolateral pouch (Fig. 171) consists of the lateral synovial wall with fat pad, the lateral malleolar surface of the talus, and the posterior surface of the lateral malleolus. The posterior talofibular ligament appears like a white tendon at the bottom of the posterolateral pouch between the tip of the lateral malleolus and the posterolateral part of the talus.

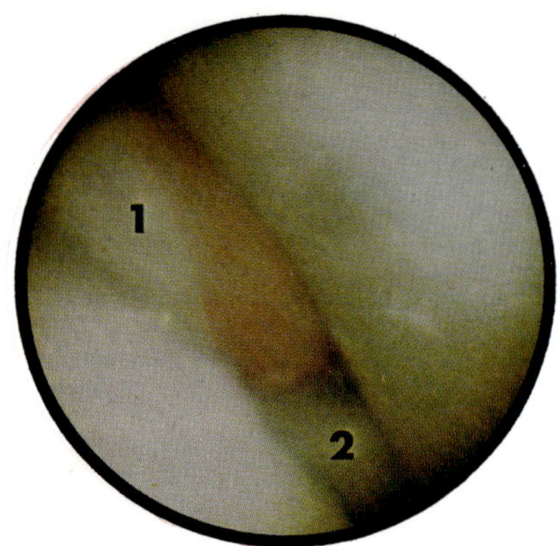

Fig. 175 Orifice of the distal tibiofibular joint with anteromedial approach. (1) Cartilaginous plica. (2) Posterior tibiofibular ligament.

The posteromedial and the posterolateral pouches increase their capacities in dorsiflexion of the ankle joint, but diminish their capacities in plantar flexion of the ankle joint.

On observing the proper talocrural joint (Fig. 172), the joint space can be slightly separated by moderately plantar flexion of the ankle joint and traction. The articular cartilage of the talus is smooth, white, or yellowish-white and glossy. The anteromedial approach provides a better view for examining the whole joint space of the proper talocrural joint.

The medial talomalleolar joint space (Fig. 173) can be slightly widened by valgus stress in plantar flexed ankle joint. At the bottom of the medial talomalleolar joint, the fibers of the deltoid ligament can sometimes be inspected under the synovial membrane.

The joint space of the talofibular (lateral talomalleolar) joint (Fig. 174) can also be slightly separated by varus stress in plantar flexed ankle joint. The posterior talofibular ligament can be inspected obliquely existed in the posterolateral pouch through the separated talofibular joint space.

The orifice of the distal tibiofibular joint (Fig. 175) can usually be seen as a slit of arthroscopy. A cartilaginous plica at the posterior part of its orifice is often observed. The anterior and the posterior tibiofibular ligaments, transversely located at the anterior and posterior of the joint, are also observed.

TECHNIQUE FOR ARTHROSCOPY OF THE ANKLE JOINT

The technique for ankle joint arthroscopy with the No. 24 arthroscope is a simple procedure, that can obtain a good view of the interior of the ankle joint.

Sterilization of Instruments

The telescopes with light guide should be sterilized by 24 hours exposure in a formalin vapor chamber. The camera with adaptor may also be sterilized in a formalin vapor chamber, but it is recommended that the same roll of film not be sterilized more than once. Telescopes are washed with sterilized normal saline solution before use.

Anesthesia

Local anesthesia in ankle joint arthroscopy is usually adequate for outpatients. But general, spinal or epidural anesthesia is better than local anesthesia to achieve adequate muscle relaxation, which ensures smooth manipulation of the arthroscope in the joint and provides a better view of the joint cavity.

Arthroscopic Procedure

The examination is carried out in an operating room under strict aseptic procedure similar that used in joint surgery. The patient is put in a supine position, and the skin is disinfected first with 3% iodine and then with 75% alcohol, and then draped.

Ankle joint arthroscopy can be performed by four approaches, i.e., the anterior approaches (medial and lateral) and the posterior approaches (medial and lateral).

Anterior approaches: The dorsal pedis artery and the anterior joint line should be palpated. Repeated dorsiflexion and plantar flexion of the talocrural joint can help palpate the joint line. After local or other type of anesthesia is applied, the ankle joint is punctured with a 20-gauge needle at the level of the anterior joint line. Any effusion is aspirated. Through the needle, the ankle joint is then filled with normal saline solution at room temperature. Usually 10 ml to 15 ml of normal saline solution is enough to amply distend the joint capsule.

With the ankle joint in right-angle position, a trocar puncture is made into the anterior pouch of the ankle joint at the anterior joint line, either medial to the anterior tibialis tendon or lateral to the peroneus tertius tendon. With the anteromedial approach, the trocar is directed to the anterior pouch from 45° medially; with the anterolateral approach, the trocar is directed from 45° laterally. Care must be taken to avoid injury to the dorsal pedis artery. The trocar is removed and an obturator is inserted so that the operator can safely confirm a successful puncture. An irrigating tube is attached to the cock of the sheath, the obturator is removed, and the telescope is introduced into the joint through the sheath. The light guide is connected to the light unit and the light is switched on. Now everything is ready for observation of the interior of the joint.

The examination is carried out under continuous injection of normal saline solution by an assistant so that sufficient hydrostatic pressure is maintained. If another trocar puncture is made, one can use an obturator to push the villi away, irrigate the joint, or perform a punch biopsy under visualization.

The anterior pouch can be examined by moving the arthroscope to and fro, while palpating the anterior wall from outside skin and manipulating the ankle joint in dorsiflexion and plantar flexion. The articular surface of the anterior half of the talus is inspected in plantar flexion of the ankle joint.

By anteromedial approach, the arthroscope with the aid of the obturator can be brought to the anteromedial pouch, the posteromedial pouch, and the posterior pouch across the proper talocrural joint space.

The anteromedial pouch should be examined while manipulating the ankle joint in dorsiflexion, plantar flexion, and varus and valgus stress. The anterior surface and the tip of the medial malleolus, the medial synovial wall, and the anterior part of the medial malleolar surface of the talus are clearly visible. After examination of the anteromedial pouch, the arthroscope (with the aid of the obturator) is moved through the medial talomalleolar joint space to examine the posteromedial pouch.

The arthroscope cannot be moved freely when it lies in the medial talomalleolar joint space. Instead, the arthroscope is gradually retracted, and a good impression of the congruence of the medial talomalleolar joint can be gained. Occasionally the fibers of the deltoid ligament can be clearly observed.

The arthroscope is then moved to the posterior pouch across the proper talocrural joint space. Sometimes the whole course of the tibial slip of the posterior talofibular ligament can now be identified. By carefully retracting and laterally moving the arthroscope, the posterior tibiofibular ligament, the orifice of the distal tibiofibular joint with its cartilaginous plica, and the entire joint space of the proper talocrural joint become visible. During this examination, the talocrural joint cannot be dorsiflexed and any forward and lateral movement of the arthroscope in the joint space should be aided by an obturator.

By anterolateral approach, the arthroscope can be moved to the anterolateral pouch. It is always possible to observe the tip of the lateral malleolus, the lateral synovial wall, the lateral articular surface of the talus, and the anterior talofibular ligament. For a better view of the anterolateral pouch, manipulation (dorsiflexion, plantar flexion, and varus and valgus stress) of the talocrural joint must be applied during examination. In a sprained ankle, a meniscoid attaching to the anterior talofibular ligament and extending into the lateral talomalleolar (talofibular) joint space is always seen.

The compartment of the posterolateral pouch can be inspected by introducing the arthroscope into this region through the talofibular joint space. The posterior talofibular ligament can be observed, located nearly horizontally in the posterolateral pouch. The arthroscope is retracted, and the talofibular joint space can then be readily observed. To obtain a better view of the lateral talomalleolar (talofibular) joint space and posterolateral pouch, varus stress must be applied while the ankle joint is kept in moderate plantar flexion.

The anterolateral approach can also be used to examine the orifice of the distal tibiofibular joint and the proper talocrural joint. With the ankle joint in about 30° plantar flexion, the end of the arthroscope is introduced into these areas. Varus stress is usually applied during observation of the orifice of the distal tibiofibular joint.

The arthroscope can reach the posterior pouch through the anteromedial approach. However, with the anterolateral approach, it is difficult to pass the arthroscope across the proper talocrural joint space into the posterior pouch because the arthroscope may be constricted by the anterior tibiofibular ligament.

Posterior approaches: The joint should be maximally distended with normal saline solution. With the patient in prone position, a posteromedial or a posterolateral puncture is made alongside the Achilles tendon, 1 cm below the posterior joint line of the ankle joint toward the posterior joint space. The trocar should be moved forward gently and slowly to avoid injury to the neurovascular bundles.

The tibial slip of the posterior talofibular ligament, the fat pad of the posterior pouch, and the posterior part of the talocrural joint can be observed by either posteromedial or posterolateral approach. The posterior recess is rarely seen because it is very shallow and usually covered by the fat pad. The posterior part of the articular surface of the talus should be examined with the ankle joint in dorsiflexion.

The posterolateral pouch with its fat pad, the posterior talofibular ligament, and the posterior surface of the lateral malleolus are examined by the posterolateral puncture. Because the posteromedial pouch is very shallow, the entire posterior compartments can almost be observed by the posterolateral puncture.

Photography

The telescope is attached by an adaptor to the camera (Olympus OM-1) and color photographs can be taken with exposure times of one-fifteenth to one-eighth second using Ektachrome (EH) film (ASA 125). Twice intensified development of the film is necessary.

Punch Biopsy

Punch biopsy under visualization is carried out by introducing the punch from another sheath. In most cases of ankle joint arthroscopy, however, biopsy is a blind procedure. Because the biopsy punch is extremely small, multiple specimens must be obtained.

Postoperative Management

On conclusion of the examination, the ankle joint is irrigated several times with normal saline solution and the sheath is withdrawn. The puncture wound is disinfected again and an adhesive plaster is affixed. An elastic bandage is then applied. The patient is allowed to walk after recovery from anesthesia. In case of local or epidural anesthesia, the patient can go home the same day. The patient is asked to rest for 24 hours after the examination and to avoid overuse of the ankle for one week.

CASE REPORTS

From January 1975 to August 1982, arthroscopy of the ankle joint was carried out on 156 ankles of 138 patients at the Tokyo Teishin Hospital and the Teikyo University Hospital. Repeat ankle arthroscopy was done twice in five ankles, and three times in two ankles. Examined were 83 ankles of 76 male patients, and 73 ankles of 62 female. The patients' ages ranged from 6 years (juvenile rheumatoid arthritis) to 75 years (rheumatoid arthritis), with an average age of 36.7 years (males, 35.2 years; females, 38.6 years).

The clinical diagnoses are shown in the Table 19. Juvenile rheumatoid arthritis and Crohn's disease were diagnosed by the Pediatric Department, and pulmonary hypertrophic osteoarthropathy due to pulmonary cancer and Behçet's disease were diagnosed by the Medical Department.

Ankle arthroscopy was done in 98 ankles under local anesthesia (62.8%), in 34 ankles under epidural anesthesia (21.8%), in 20 ankles under lumbar anesthesia (12.8%), and in 4 ankles under general anesthesia (2.6%). Approaches used for the ankle arthroscopy are shown in the Table 20. In 67 ankles anterolateral approach was used (41.8%), in 44 ankles anteromedial approach (27.5%), and in 37 ankles combined anterolateral and anteromedial approaches (23.1%). The posterior approaches were used only in selected cases.

Most patients with sprained ankles complained of persistent, mild pain in the ankle on certain movements—no pain on walking, but pain with tenderness over the anterodistal area of the lateral malleolus and/or pain in the anterior joint line of the ankle on dorsiflexion. Occasionally a patient complained of medial malleolar pain. Ankle arthroscopy was done to confirm the etiology of the persistent pain. In patients with sprained ankles, 18 meniscoids were observed, revealing five cases of avulsion or injury of the meniscoid, six cases associated with partial rupture of the anterior talofibular ligament, and seven cases of articular cartilage ulcer or chondral fracture.

Case 1 A 42-year-old man with left ankle sprain (Fig. 176).

The patient fell down on the road and suffered a left ankle sprain on December 15, 1976. He presented with complaints of the left ankle swelling and pain on December 17, 1976. Anterolateral approach arthroscopy of the left ankle joint was done on December 24, 1976, under local anesthesia, revealing proliferation of villi in the anterior joint cavity, partial rupture of the posterior attachment of the meniscoid, and uneven articular surface of the talus. Partial rupture of the anterior talofibular ligament was also observed by varus stress of the ankle.

Case 2 A 29-year-old man with left ankle sprain (Fig. 177).

The patient suffered a left ankle sprain in a Rugby game on February 20, 1978. Physical examination of the left ankle at first visit on the same day revealed swelling, tenderness, and limitation of motion of the left ankle joint. Anterolateral approach arthroscopy of the left ankle joint was carried out on June 9, 1978, under local anesthesia, because of persistent pain in the left ankle. Proliferation of hyperemic villi, avulsion of the

Table 19 Cases examined by arthroscopy of the ankle joint and their clinical conditions

Clinical condition	Male				Female				Total	
	Right	Left	Both	Joints	Right	Left	Both	Joints	Patients	Joints
Pain in a joint	2	2	0	4	2	5	0	7	11	11
Sprain	10	16	0	26	8	6	0	14	40	40
Dislocation	1	1	0	2	0	0	0	0	2	2
Intraarticular fracture										
Lateral malleolus	2	2	1	6	1	1	0	2	7	8
Medial malleolus	3	2	0	5	3	0	0	3	8	8
Bilateral malleoli	3	0	0	3	0	1	0	1	4	4
Talus	2	1	0	3	0	0	0	0	3	3
Tibia	0	1	0	1	0	0	0	0	1	1
Extraarticular fracture										
Calcaneus	2	0	0	2	0	0	0	0	2	2
Tibia, fibula	2	0	0	2	1	0	0	1	3	3
Loose body	2	1	0	3	3	2	0	5	8	8
Osteochondritis dissecans (talus)	1	0	0	1	0	0	1	2	2	3
Nonspecific arthritis	3	1	0	4	2	1	0	3	7	7
Osteoarthritis	0	2	0	2	0	0	3	6	5	8
Rheumatoid arthritis	2	2	2	8	3	6	7	23	22	31
Juvenile rheumatoid arthritis	0	0	0	0	1	0	0	1	1	1
Gouty arthritis	1	1	2	6	0	0	0	0	4	6
Pulmonary hypertrophic osteoarthropathy	0	0	1	2	0	0	0	0	1	2
Crohn's disease	0	0	0	0	0	1	0	1	1	1
Behçet's disease	0	0	0	0	1	0	0	1	1	1
Suppurative arthritis	0	0	1	2	2	0	0	2	3	4
Traumatic arthritis	0	1	0	1	1	0	0	1	2	2
Total	36	33	7	83	28	23	11	73	138	156

Right=The number of patients whose right ankle was examined. Left=Left ankle examined. Both=Both right and left ankles examined.
Joints=The number of times of ankle joint arthroscopy: some ankles were examined repeatedly.

Table 20 The number of approaches for arthroscopy of the ankle joint by clinical condition

Clinical condition	Joints	Approaches								Total
		AL	AM	AL+AM	AL+PM	AL+PL	PM	AM+PM	PL+PM	
Pain in a joint	11	6	1	2	1	0	1	0	0	11
Sprain	40	24	11	5	0	0	0	0	0	40
Dislocation	2	1	2	0	0	0	0	0	0	3
Intraarticular fracture										
Lateral malleolus	8	8	0	0	0	0	0	0	0	8
Medial malleolus	8	1	2	4	0	1	0	0	0	8
Bilateral malleolus	4	1	0	3	0	0	0	0	0	4
Talus	3	1	0	2	0	0	0	0	0	3
Tibia	1	0	1	0	0	0	0	0	0	1
Extraarticular fracture										
Calcaneus	2	1	0	1	0	0	0	0	0	2
Tibia, fibula	3	0	2	1	0	0	0	0	0	3
Loose body	8	4	1	0	0	0	1	1	1	8
Nonspecific arthritis	7	3	2	2	0	0	0	0	0	7
Osteoarthritis	8	4	1	2	0	0	0	1	0	8
Rheumatoid arthritis	31	8	15	4	0	0	3	2	0	32
Juvenile rheumatoid arthritis	1	0	1	0	0	0	0	0	0	1
Gouty arthritis	6	2	3	1	0	0	0	0	0	6
Pulmonary hypertrophic osteopathy	2	1	1	0	0	0	0	0	0	2
Crohn's disease	1	0	0	1	0	0	0	0	0	1
Behçet's disease	1	0	0	1	0	0	0	0	0	1
Suppurative arthritis	4	0	0	4	0	0	0	0	0	4
Traumatic arthritis	2	0	0	2	0	0	0	0	0	2
Osteochondritis dissecans (talus)	3	2	1	2	0	0	0	0	0	5
Total	156	67	44	37	1	1	5	4	1	160

AM=Anteromedial. AL=Anterolateral. PM=Posteromedial. PL=Posterolateral.

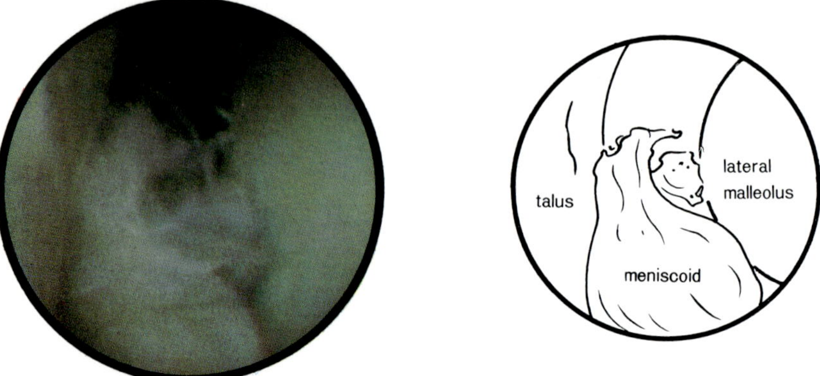

Fig. 176 Case 1. A 42-year-old man with left ankle sprain. Partial rupture of the posterior attachment of the meniscoid, anterolateral approach.

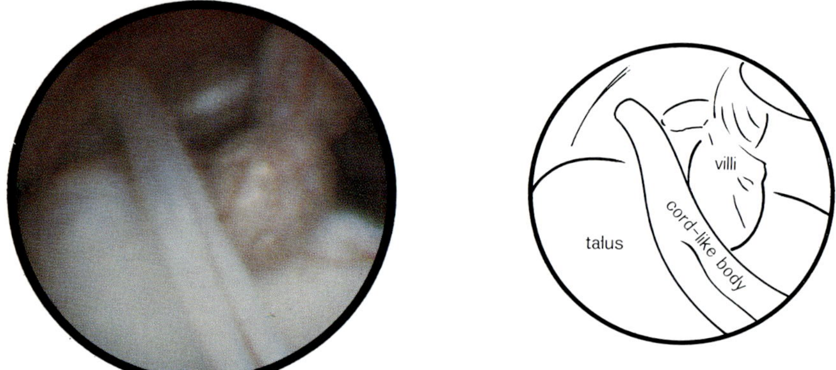

Fig. 177 Case 2. A 29-year-old man with left ankle sprain. A cord-like body, anterolateral approach.

articular cartilage of the talus, a big cartilaginous anterolateral synovial plica, and an anteromedial synovial plica were seen. A cord-like body was observed extending from the anteromedial synovial plica to the anterolateral wall of the ankel joint.

Case 3 A 20-year-old man with right ankle sprain (Fig. 178).

The patient sustained a traffic accident with a distortion of his right ankle on December 16, 1976. His first visit the next day revealed tenderness over the right lateral malleolus. Anterolateral approach arthroscopy of the right ankle on December 22, 1976, under local anesthesia, revealed an articular cartilage ulcer of the talus and disastasis of the distal tibiofibular joint.

Case 4 A 20-year-old woman with left ankle sprain (Fig. 179).

The patient sustained left ankle sprain while skiing in January 1977. Her first visit on August 17, 1977, revealed tenderness over both the medial and lateral malleoli of her left ankle. Anteromedial and anterolateral approach arthroscopy of the left ankle was performed on August 30, 1977, under local anesthesia. An avulsion of the lateral malleous with pannus-like tissue was seen. Proliferation of villi with articular cartilage was also observed. The posterior talofibular ligament was seen to run more obliquely than ordinarily. The capillaries on the tibial slip were clearly observed.

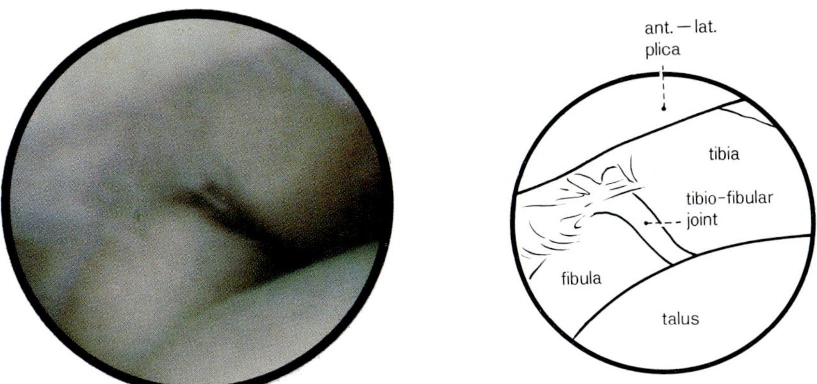

Fig. 178 Case 3. A 20-year-old man with right ankle sprain. Widened tibiofibular joint, anterolateral approach.

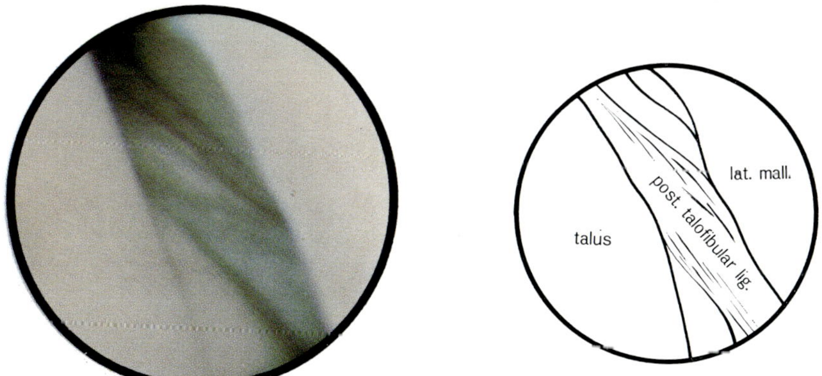

Fig. 179 Case 4. A 20-year-old woman with left ankle sprain. Posterior talofibular ligament, anterolateral approach.

Case 5 A 52-year-old woman with left ankle sprain (Fig. 180).

The patient fell from stairs with a resulting of sprain of her left ankle on July 12, 1975. She presented on December 23, 1976, with a complaint of motion pain in her left ankle. Physical examination revealed mild swelling, tenderness on the anterior talotibial joint line, and motion pain of the left ankle. Anterolateral approach arthroscopy of the left ankle on January 17, 1977, under epidural anesthesia, revealed an articular cartilage fracture of the tibia, partial rupture of the anterior talofibular ligament, and a meniscoid injury.

Case 6 A 29-year-old man with left ankle sprain (Fig. 181).

On April 29, 1977, the patient stumbled and fell forward during a baseball game, with a feeling of anterior displacement of his left distal tibia. His first visit on July 14, 1977, revealed pain but a negative anterior drawer test on the left ankle joint. Anteromedial approach arthroscopy of the left ankle joint on August 2, 1977, under local anesthesia, revealed a rupture of the tibial slip, villi proliferation, and articular surface ulcer of the talus.

Case 7 A 6-year-old girl with avulsion fracture of the left lateral malleolus (Fig. 182).

The patient suffered a left ankle sprain in a fall one year before presentation to our department. Her first visit on September 8, 1975, revealed a fracture of the left lateral

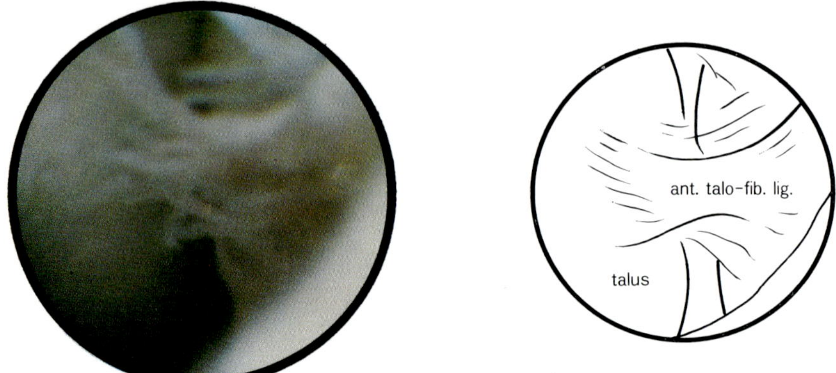

Fig. 180 Case 5. A 52-year-old woman with left ankle sprain. Partial rupture of the anterior talofibular ligament, anterolateral approach.

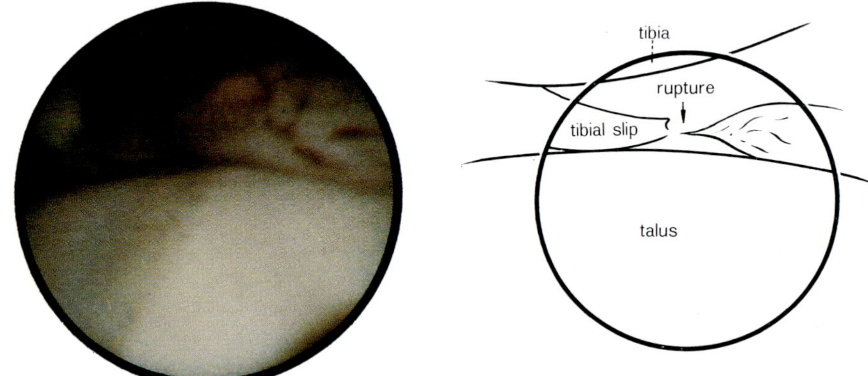

Fig. 181 Case 6. A 29-year-old man with left ankle sprain. Rupture of the tibial slip, anteromedial approach.

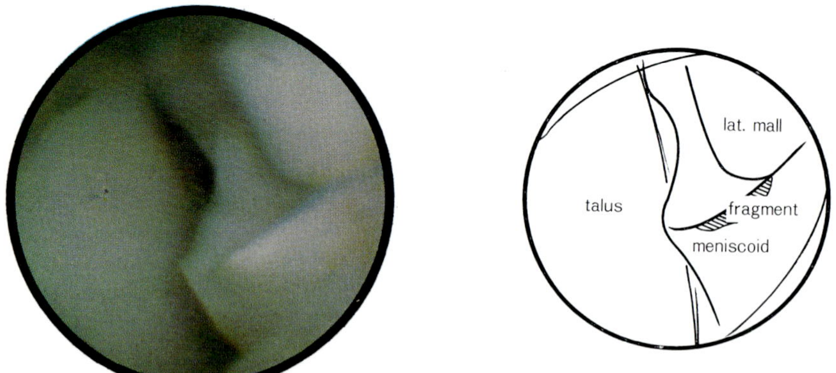

Fig. 182 Case 7. A 6-year-old girl with avulsion fracture of the left lateral malleolus, anterolateral approach.

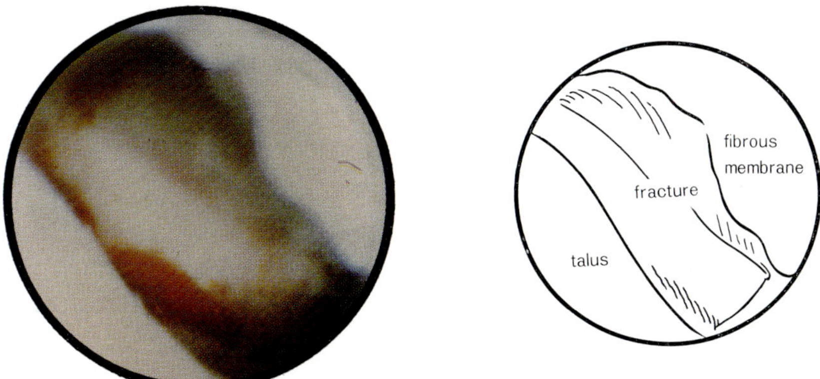

Fig. 183 Case 8. A 23-year-old man with fracture of the medial malleolus on the right, anteromedial approach.

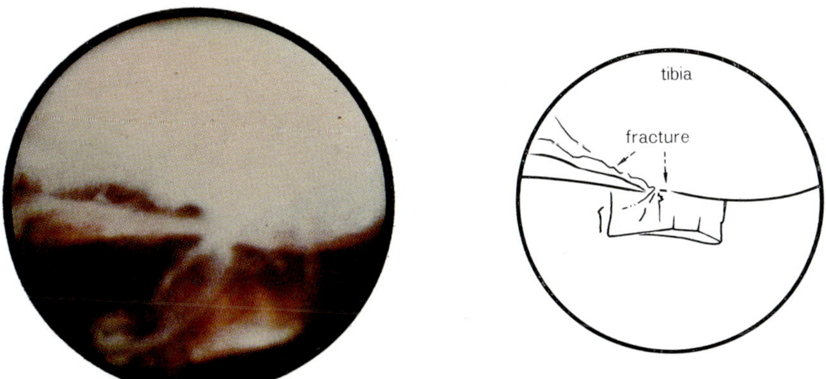

Fig. 184 Case 9. A 28-year-old man with intraarticular fracture of the left tibia, anteromedial approach.

malleolus on a X-ray plain film. A belt-like tissue with its fracture fragment surrounding the lateral malleolus was seen on air arthrography of the ankle joint. Anterolateral approach arthroscopy of the left ankle joint on September 6, 1976, under spinal anesthesia, revealed a belt-like tissue—same as the arthrographic finding—which was excised by arthrotomy. One of the origins of the meniscoid was suggested by this case.

Case 8 A 23-year-old man with fractures of the right medial and lateral malleoli (Fig. 183). The patient twisted his right ankle in a baseball game on August 28, 1976. The above clinical diagnosis was made at his first visit on August 31, 1976. Arthroscopy of the right ankle was carried out via the anteromedial and anterolateral approaches under epidural anesthesia. Figure 183 shows the fracture of the medial malleolus in the right ankle.

Case 9 A 28-year-old man with fracture of the left distal tibia (Figs. 184 and 185). The patient fell while skiing on February 21, 1977. His first visit on February 25, 1977, revealed swelling, tenderness, local warmth, and limitation of motion of the left ankle joint. Anteromedial approach arthroscopy of the left ankle on February 28, 1977, under local anesthesia, revealed osteochondral fracture of the tibial surface and articular fracture of the talus.

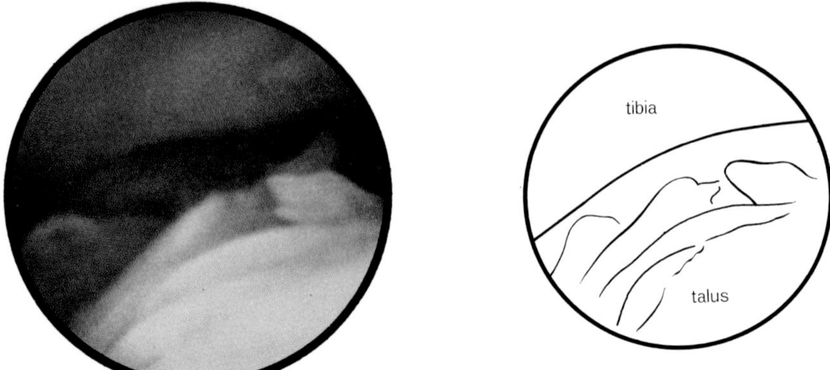

Fig. 185 Case 9. Cartilage fracture of the left talus, anteromedial approach.

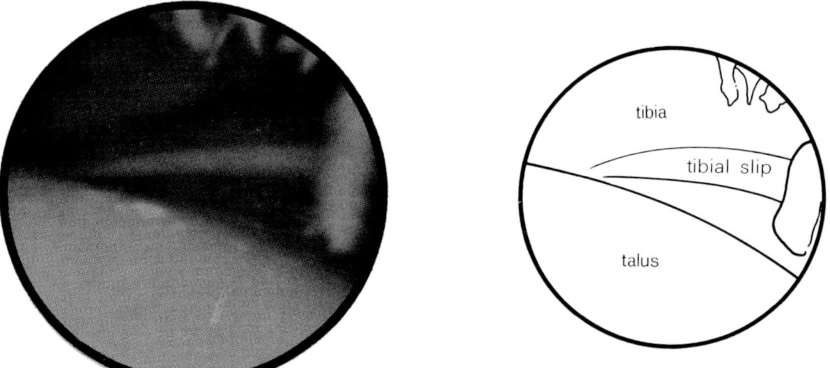

Fig. 186 Case 10. A 62-year-old woman with osteoarthritis on the right ankle. Tibial slip, anteromedial approach.

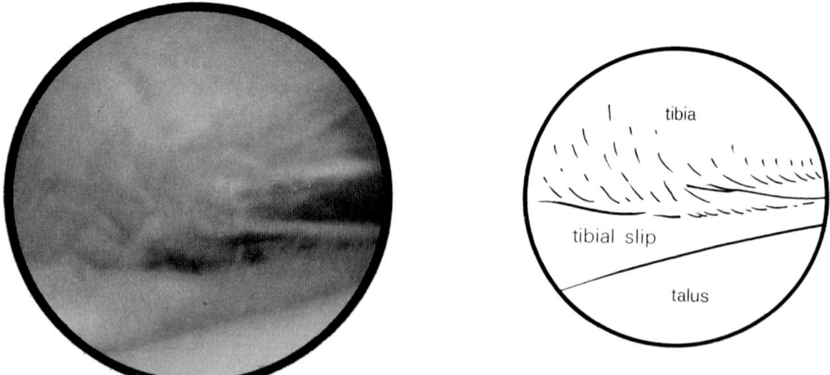

Fig. 187 Case 11. A 66-year-old woman with osteoarthritis in the right ankle. Tibial slip, anteromedial approach.

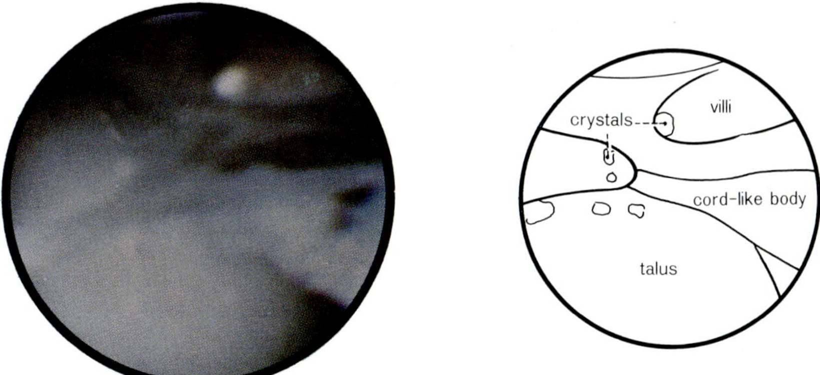

Fig. 188 Case 12. A 21-year-old man with gouty arthritis in the left ankle, anterolateral approach.

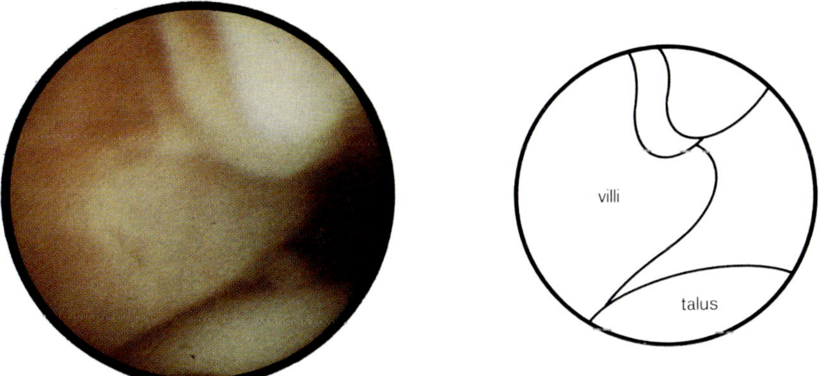

Fig. 189 Case 13. Left ankle of 9-year-old girl with Crohn's disease. Proliferation of villi, anteromedial approach.

Case 10 A 62-year-old woman with osteoarthritis of the right ankle joint (Fig. 186). The patient had had varus deformity of the both ankle joints with occasional pain for ten years. Her first visit on February 5, 1976, revealed swelling, mild local warmth, and varus deformities on both ankle joints. Arthroscopy of the left ankle joint was carried out with combined anteromedial and anterolateral approaches on January 26, 1977, under local anesthesia. The tibial slip was observed, as shown in Figure 186.

Case 11 A 66-year-old woman with osteoarthritis of the right ankle joint (Fig. 187). The patient complained of pain in the both ankles for two years. Her first visit on January 11, 1977, revealed varus deformities with swelling and pain on motion of both ankles. Anteromedial approach arthroscopy of both ankles performed on January 28, 1977, under local anesthesia, revealed fibrous change of the tibial slip surface and the articular cartilage of the tibia of the right ankle.

Case 12 A 21-year-old man with gouty arthritis in the left ankle joint (Fig. 188). The patient had had attacks of gouty arthritis of both ankles for several months. His first visit on November 21, 1976, revealed pain, swelling, and local warmth in the left ankle. Arthroscopy of the left ankle via the anterolateral approach was carried out on December 27, 1977, under local anesthesia, because of repeat attacks. Hyperemic

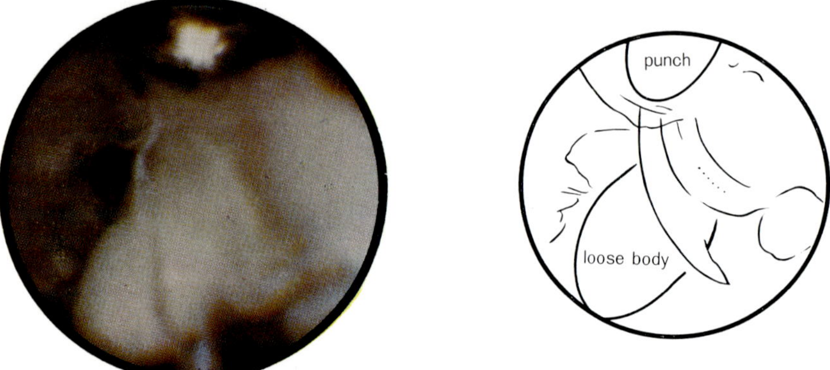

Fig. 190 Case 14. A 33-year-old man with a loose body in the left ankle, anterolateral approach.

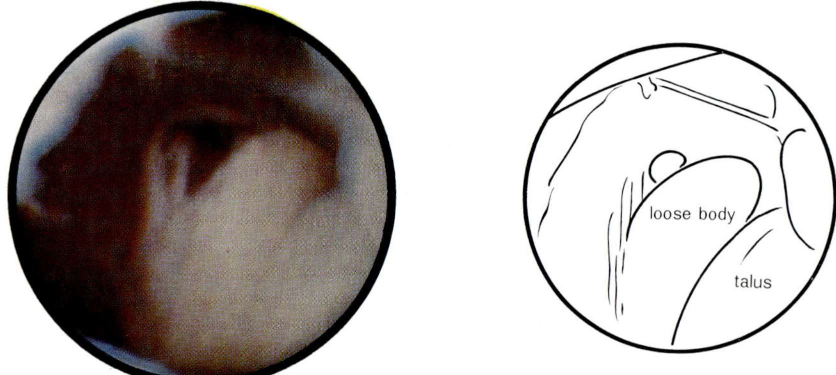

Fig. 191 Case 15. A 35-year-old man with a loose body in the posterior pouch of the right ankle, posterolateral approach.

swollen villi with whitish spot crystal on their tips and precipitation of the crystal on the articular cartilage surface were observed.

Case 13 A 9-year-old girl with Crohn's disease (Fig. 189).

The patient complained of left ankle pain after an athletic meeting on October 3, 1976. Her first visit on October 20, 1976, revealed tenderness in her left ankle. Anteromedial approach arthroscopy of the left ankle was carried out on March 1, 1977, under local anesthesia, because of the repeat attacks of pain and swelling. Granulomatous villi filled the whole joint cavity.

Case 14 A 33-year-old man with a loose body in the left ankle (Fig. 190).

The patient had a left ankle sprain in a baseball game five years before presentation. In August 1979, the patient again sprained the same ankle. Two months later, the patient noted a click of the left ankle on standing after sitting or riding a bicycle. His first visit on November 13, 1979, revealed a click on supination with dorsiflexion and plantar flexion of the ankle. A plain X-ray film of the ankle revealed a loose body in the left ankle. Arthroscopy of the left ankle via the anterolateral approach under epidural anesthesia was carried out on April 24, 1980. The loose body was found in the anterior pouch of the ankle, and was removed under arthroscopic visualization.

Case 15 A 35-year-old man with a loose body in the right ankle (Fig. 191).
The patient had violent hyperplantar flexion of the right ankle during a baseball game in the summer of 1975. He experienced the same stress of hyperplantar flexion of his right ankle during work on March 26, 1976. Thereafter, pain in his right ankle persisted. His first visit on January 9, 1980, revealed tenderness around the lateral malleolus, and a loose body was seen on plain X-ray film. Under epidural anesthesia, arthroscopy of the right ankle via the posterolateral approach revealed a loose body attached on the synovium of the posterior pouch. The loose body articulated with the lateral tubercle of the talus, which was removed by arthrotomy. The distal tibiofibular joint line was also observed via posteromedial approach arthroscopy.

10

Arthroscopy of the Temporomandibular Joint

INTRODUCTION

Since the development of the Watanabe No. 24 arthroscope, arthroscopy of the temporomandibular joint (TM joint) has been possible. In 1975, Ohnishi reported the clinical introduction of arthroscopic technique for the TM joint. In 1980, Kino reported the morphological observation of the superior articular cavity of the TM joint, relating to the endoscopic findings in fresh cadavers. In 1981, the authors reported the arthroscopic anatomy and arthroscopic approaches of the TM joint, based on a fundamental arthroscopic study in human cadavers. Kino et al. also studied the morphology of the superior articular cavity in human TM joint and described some clinical terminology for arthroscopic findings. Ohnishi described the clinical usefulness of arthroscopy for TM joint diseases, and in our laboratory the detailed regional anatomy correlating to the arthroscopic anatomy of human cadavers was investigated proposing new nomenclature for regional anatomic and arthroscopic descriptions of the human TM joint, and also the arthroscopic anatomy and histology of human cadaver TM joints was studied in 1982, respectively.

Arthroscopy of the TM joint using the Watanabe No. 24 arthroscope has developed into a clinically useful method.

ANATOMY OF THE TEMPOROMANDIBULAR JOINT

The TM joint consists of an upper gliding joint, a lower hinge joint, and an intervening articular disk. The bony components of the TM joint are the temporal bone and the mandible, of which the bony surface is not covered by hyaline cartilage, but by fibrocartilage. As the right and left TM joints are situated on the bilateral end of the mandible, the twin TM joints function together harmoniously and are responsible for complex mandibular movements against the cranium.

The articular cavity is divided into the superior and inferior articular cavities by the articular disk. The anterior portion of the articular disk is interwoven with the sphenomeniscus portion of the lateral pterygoid muscle, and the posterior structure of the articular disk is transient to the retrodiscal fat pad. The bilateral part of the articular disk is firmly attached downward to the medial and lateral poles of the mandibular head.

The lateral and medial capsules are loose and thin membranes that cover the temporal bone, the circumference of the mandibular fossa, the articular tubercle, and below to the mandibular neck. The anterior and posterior capsules cannot be clearly identified because of the much more complicated adjacent structures such as the muscles and the retrodiscal fat pad. The lateral ligament directly reinforces the TM joint. The other two accessory ligaments are attached only to the mandible and the cranium. These are shown in Figure 192.

ARTHROSCOPIC ANATOMY

The articular cavity is separated into a temporodiscal interspace and a condylodiscal interspace, which can be subdivided arthroscopically into the synovial pouches and the intermediate spaces (the space between the articular surfaces). These are shown in Figure 193.

The intraarticular inner surface consists of the articular surface and the synovial membrane. The transitional zones of these features are not clear, but they are distinguishable. The articular surface of the temporal bone consists of the surface of the mandibular fossa and the articular tubercle. The articular surface of the mandible is the surface of the mandibular head. The articular surface of the articular disk is the central part of the upper and lower surface plus the peripheral zone. The synovial membrane lines the inner surface of the articular cavity other than the articular surfaces, which can be clearly observed in the anteroposterior reflectional zone. The surface of the synovial membrane is altered by formation of the synovial folds through positional change of the articular disk following movement of the mandible.

The upper surface of the articular disk shows a contour resembling a lying sigmoid shape. It consists of two parts: the discal eminence, or the posterior highest portion; and the flat portion, or the anterior sloping portion. The lower surface of the articular disk is concave and is referred to as the discal fossa.

The temporodiscal interspace (superior articular cavity) can be subdivided into the upper anterior and upper posterior synovial pouches, and the higher and lower intermediate spaces. The higher intermediate space is the space between the articular surfaces of the mandibular fossa and the articular disk, and the lower intermediate space is the space between the articular surface of the articular tubercle and the articular disk. The upper posterior synovial pouch begins at the posterior border of the discal articular surface, slightly behind the discal eminence and above the posterior rim of the articular surface of the mandibular fossa. The medial and lateral synovial wall and the articular disk form a groove. The articular disk firmly attaches downward to the medial and lateral poles of the mandibular head, where the groove is referred to as the medial and lateral paradiscal synovial groove.

The condylodiscal interspace (inferior articular cavity) can be also subdivided into the lower anterior and lower posterior synovial pouches between the intermediate space. The intermediate space in this cavity is a minute space between the articular surfaces of the mandibular head and the articular disk. In the deepest portion of the lower posterior synovial pouch, the anteriorly located condylar surface and the posteriorly located synovial surface face each other very closely. They form a deep narrow groove without the synovial reflection seen in the upper posterior synovial pouch. The articular space is narrower and less movable than the superior articular cavity. These are shown in Figures 193 and 194.

APPROACHES AND VISIBLE FIELDS

Avoiding injury to important structures adjacent to the TM joint is essential in considering arthroscopic approach. In the TM joint, the operator should consider the facial nerve, the superficial temporal branch of the auriculotemporal nerve, the superficial temporal artery

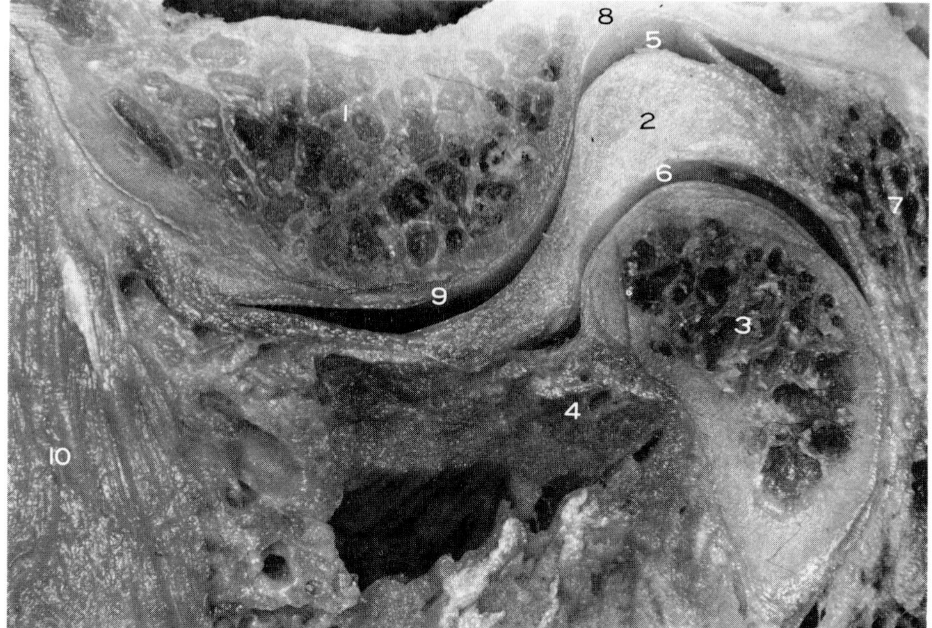

a

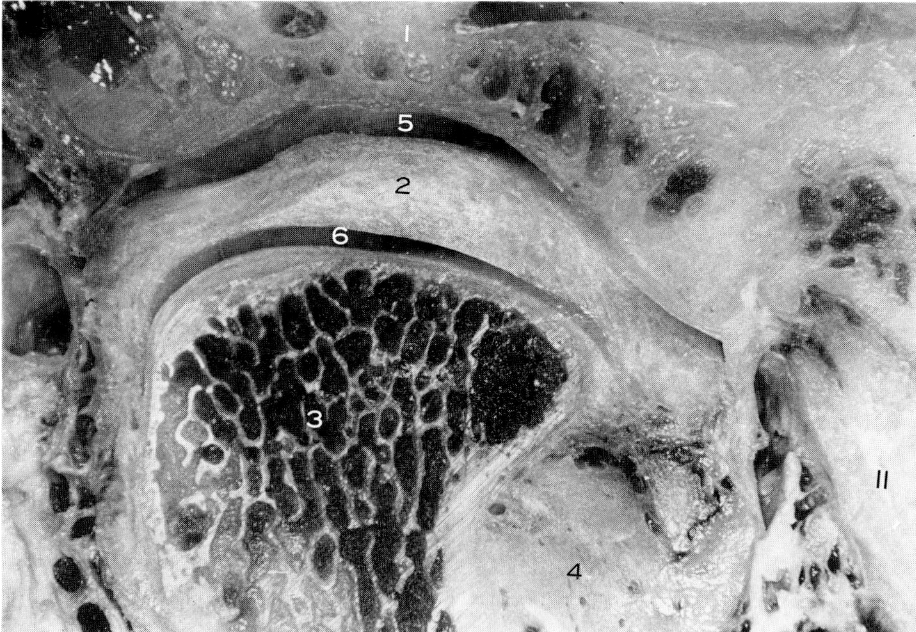

b

Fig. 192 Temporomandibular joint (Murakami and Hoshino, unpublished). (a) Sagittal section of the left joint. (b) Coronal section of the right TM joint. (1) Temporal bone. (2) Articular disk. (3) Head of the mandible. (4) Lateral pterygoid muscle. (5) Superior articular cavity. (6) Inferior articular cavity. (7) Retrodiscal fat pad. (8) Mandibular fossa. (9) Articular tubercle. (10) Masseter muscle. (11) Levator veli palatini muscle.

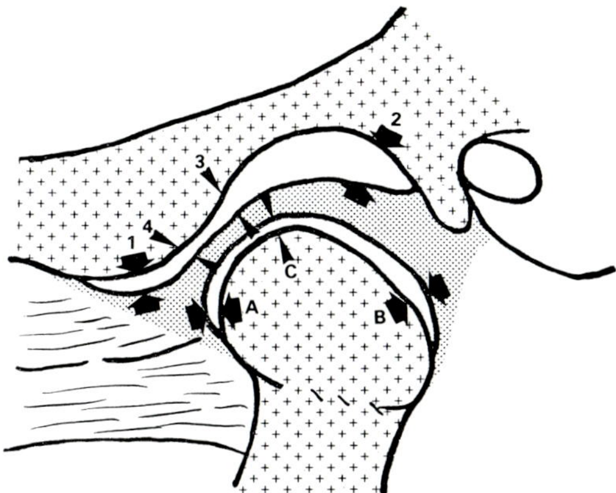

Fig. 193 Arthroscopic anatomy. Subdivision of the intraarticular space. *Temporodiscal interspace (superior articular cavity)*: (1) Upper anterior synovial pouch. (2) Upper posterior synovial pouch. (3) Higher intermediate space. (4) Lower intermediate space. *Condylodiscal interspace (inferior articular cavity)*: (A) Lower anterior synovial pouch. (B) Lower posterior synovial pouch. (C) Intermediate space.

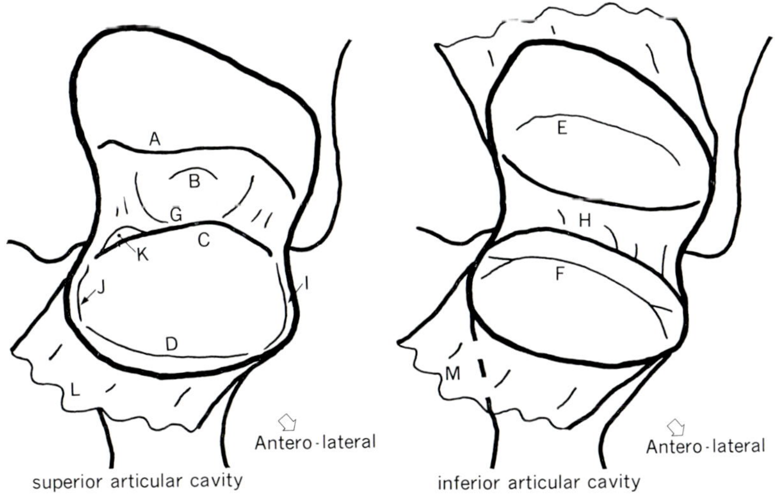

Fig. 194 Arthroscopic anatomy of the left TM joint, opened from the front toward the back. *Temporal bone:* (A) Articular tubercle. (B) Mandibular fossa. *Articular disk:* (C) Discal eminence. (D) Flat portion. (E) Discal fossa. *Mandible:* (F) Head of the mandible. *Synovial membrane:* (G) In upper posterior synovial pouch. (H) In lower posterior synovial pouch. (I) Lateral paradiscal synovial groove. (J) Medial paradiscal synovial groove. (K) Tongue-like synovial plica. *Lateral pterygoid muscle:* (L) Sphenomeniscus portion. (M) Lower portion.

and vein, and the parotid gland. The operator should also focus attention on dangerous conditions such as intraarticular damage of the articular cartilage and the articular disk caused by arthroscopic examination. The three approaches described below are clinically useful (Fig. 195).

Inferolateral Approach

In the jaw opening, the mandibular head is rotated and glided downward and forward.

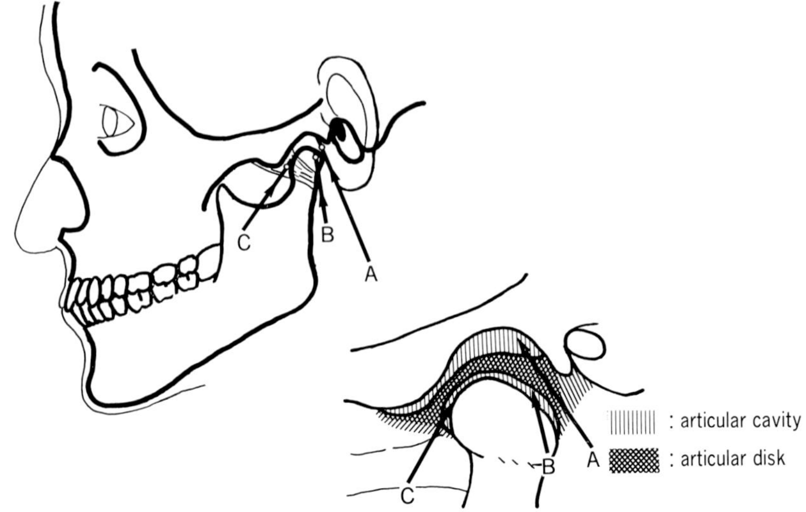

Fig. 195 Arthroscopic approaches. (A) Inferolateral approach. (B) Posterolateral approach. (C) Anterolateral approach.

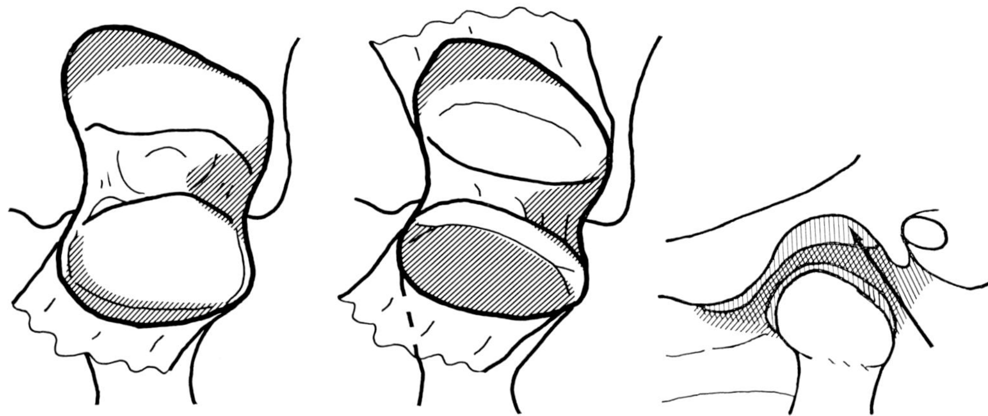

Fig. 196 Visible fields by inferolateral approach. Dark areas are difficult to observe.

The triangular pouch can be palpated in front of the tragus, which is bordered superiorly by the mandibular fossa, anteroinferiorly by the dorsal surface of the mandibular head, and posteriorly by the external acoustic meatus. This pouch is the entry point. To avoid the superficial temporal artery, the artery should be palpated before insertion of the trocar. The tip of the inserting trocar is directed anteriorly toward the coronal plane at an angle of 20°, and superiorly toward the horizontal plane at an angle 20°. This method allows penetration to the superior articular cavity. It is important for exact insertion to first feel the temporal articular surface with the top of the blunt trocar. For the inferior articular cavity, the top of the trocar is oriented downward to the dorsal surface of the mandibular head. Following touch of the blunt trocar to the dorsal surface of the condyle, the tip of trocar is inserted along the condylar surface. These approaches and their visible fields are shown in Figures 196 and 197. The upper anterior synovial pouch, and the medial paradiscal

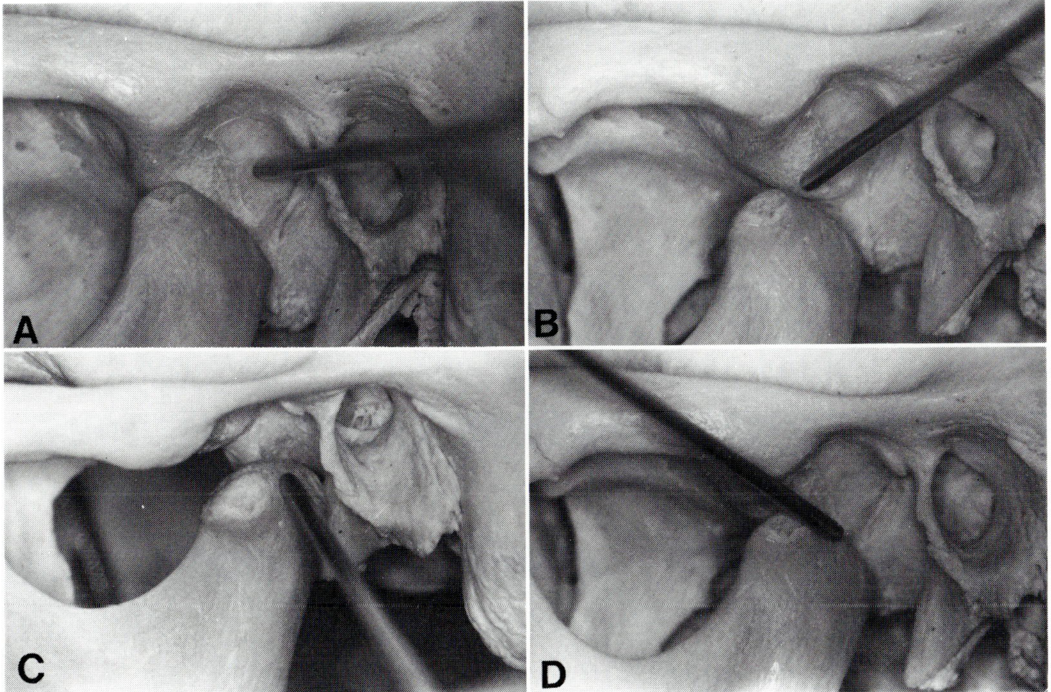

Fig. 197 Inferolateral approach. *Temporodiscal interspace (superior articular cavity)*: (A) The blunt trocar is pointed toward the mandibular fossa for observation of the upper posterior synovial pouch. (B) The blunt trocar is then moved toward the articular tubercle for observation of the higher intermediate space. *Condylodiscal interspace (inferior articular cavity)*: (C) The tip of the blunt trocar is pointed toward the lateral posterior surface of the mandibular head. (D) The trocar is moved along the posterior surface of the mandibular head for observation of the lower posterior synovial pouch.

synovial groove are occasionally difficult to observe in the temporodiscal interspace. The lower anterior synovial pouch and the lateral part of the lower posterior synovial pouch are also difficult to observe in the condylodiscal interspace.

Posterolateral Approach

This approach is suitable for observation of the lower posterior synovial pouch. In the jaw opening, the trocar puncture is made at the one fingerbreadth frontal from the tragus in the triangular pouch (as same in inferolateral approach). The top of the trocar is directed against the lateral posterior surface of the mandibular head. Condylar movement should be confirmed with the blunt trocar. Part of the synovial membrane in the lower posterior synovial pouch, a part of the discal fossa, and the posterior condylar surface can be examined as shown in Figure 198.

Anterolateral Approach

This approach is suitable for observation of the lower anterior synovial pouch However, it is not so easy as compared with the above two approaches. The articular tubercle and mandibular head should be exactly palpated with repeated jaw movements in various directions. The trocar should be inserted at the point in front of the mandibular lateral

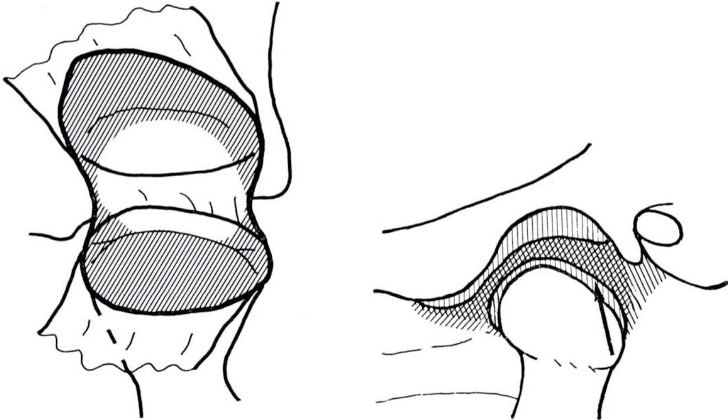

Fig. 198 Visible fields by posterolateral approach.

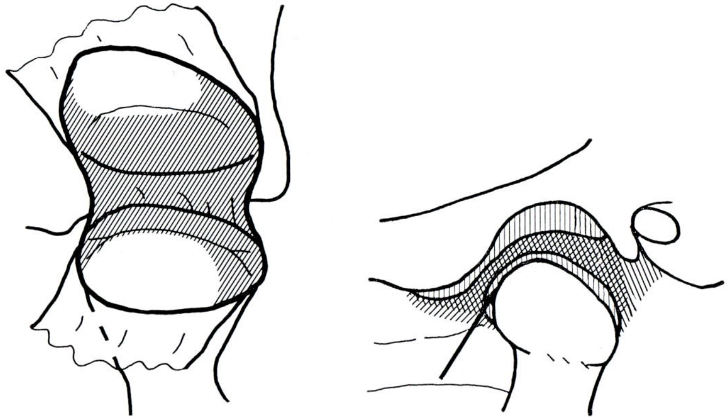

Fig. 199 Visible fields by anterolateral approach.

pole and immediately below the articular tubercle under the biting position. Through the lateral ligament, the trocar is inserted into the lower anterior synovial pouch along the anterior surface of the mandibular head, with the tip of the trocar directed toward the lateral anterior part of the mandibular head. Only the lower anterior synovial pouch is visible, as shown in Figure 199.

CLINICAL ARTHROSCOPY

Basic Technique

There is no difference in procedure for arthroscopy of the TM joint as compared with that for the other small joints. However, as mentioned above, the TM joint is so narrow that the superior and inferior articular cavities cannot be distended sufficiently to allow satisfactory intraarticular manipulation. It is very important to preserve the articular disk and the articular cartilage under intraarticular manipulation, so the following points should be considered both before and during the operation.

1. The joint space should be fully distended for the trocar puncture by injecting 2 ml to 4 ml of normal saline into the superior articular cavity, and 1 ml to 3 ml of normal

saline into the inferior articular cavity. (Usually, the first injection may be replaced with anesthetics.)

2. Use of the sharp trocar should be limited to the skin insertion and capsular puncture.
3. Intraarticular manipulation should be done carefully and gently using the blunt trocar.
4. The articular space should be expanded during arthroscopy by pressure of normal saline, which should be supplied via an infusion syringe by an assistant.

Anesthesia

Arthroscopic examination under general anesthesia is, needless to say possible, but it does not facilitate easy positioning of the mandible. Intraarticular anesthesia is more favorable for arthroscopy of the TM joint because the patient can position and move the jaw according to the operator's instructions. At first, infiltration anesthesia with 0.5% lidocaine should be applied on the entry point of the skin. After that, a 21-gauge needle is inserted into the objective joint space, and the articular space is filled with 2% lidocaine. This method provides an anesthetic duration of about one hour.

Preparation and Other Considerations

Arthroscopy is carried out in the outpatient operating room with the patient sitting on the dental chair. A stabilized head rest that permits free movement of the TM joint is important. There should be no limitations on jaw movement. Preoperative shaving and disinfection are done in the usual manner. Clear photography is possible with arthroscopy, as well as punch biopsy and other procedures done through the outer sheath.

Normal Arthroscopic View (Fig. 200)

The single puncture approach does not permit whole-area observation of the articular cavity of the TM joint. Even with combinations of the three approaches mentioned above, the following areas are difficult to observe: the medial paradiscal synovial groove, and the intermediate space in the inferior articular cavity.

The articular surface usually appears smooth, avascular, and shiny with a ivory-whitish tinge. Discal articular surface is more whitish and compact than the bony articular surface. Neither articular surface changes its view with jaw movement. As compared with these appearances, the inner surface of the synovial membrane appears softer and more flexible, less shiny with a velvet-like texture, and has a translucent vascular pattern.

Significantly different from other structures, the surface of the synovial membrane is altered by the formation of synovial folds through positional change of the articular disk following movement of the mandible. These synovial folds are clearly visualized in the upper posterior synovial pouch. Occasionally, some synovial folds—called synovial plica—may persist on the surface of the synovial membrane, as seen in the synovial pouch and groove. As compared with the upper posterior synovial pouch, the synovial membrane in the lower posterior synovial pouch looks more vascularized due to the blood vessels of the retrodiscal fat pad present deep to the synovial membrane. Therefore, the synovial membrane in this pouch looks softer and more flexible. However, the synovial fold as in the upper synovial pouch cannot be observed, although a pad-like cushion can be visualized.

CLINICAL CASES

Case 1 A 37-year-old woman with subacute traumatic arthritis of the TM joint (Fig. 201).

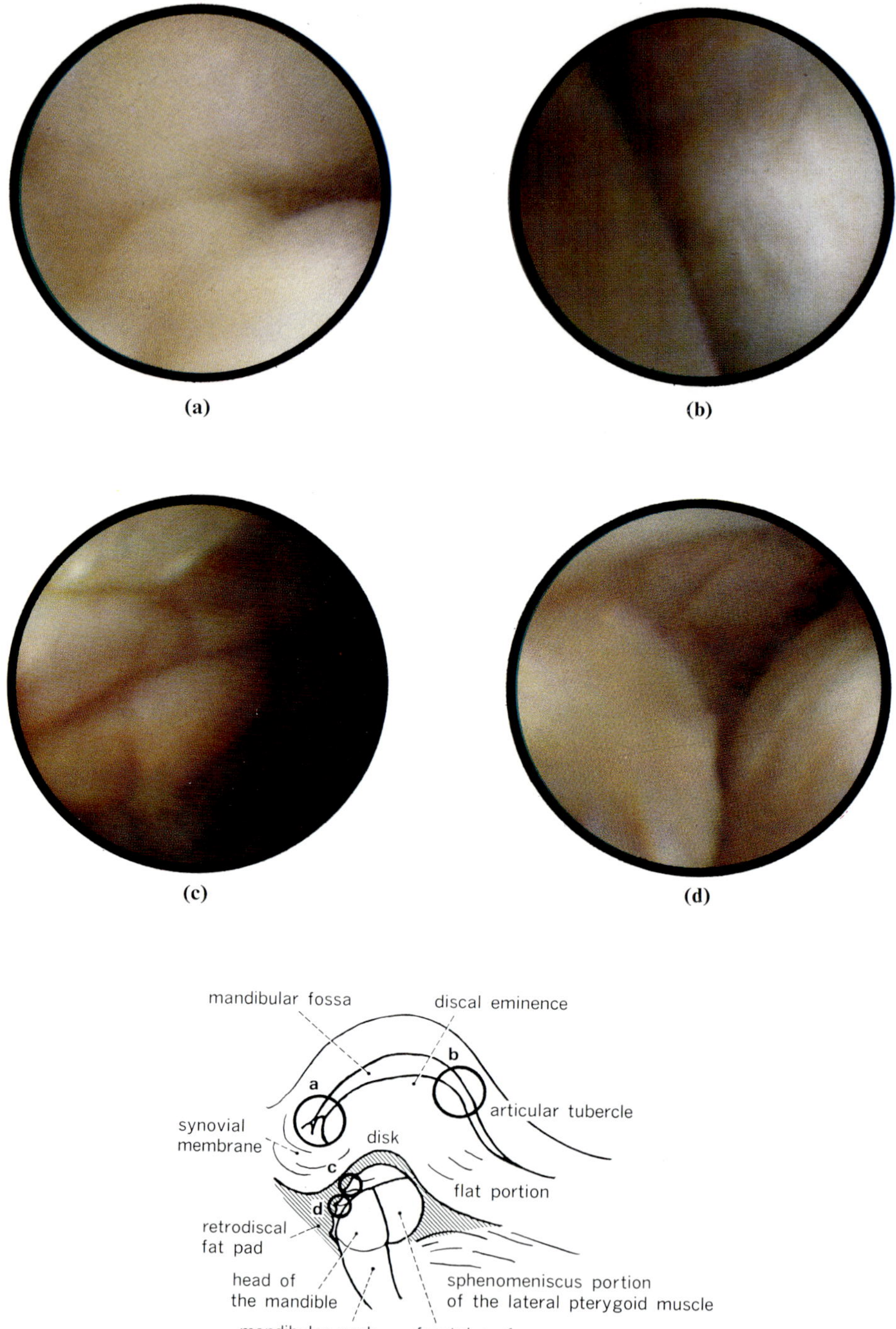

Fig. 200 Normal arthroscopic view in human cadaver. (a) Upper posterior synovial pouch. (b) Higher intermediate space. (c, d) Lower posterior synovial pouch.

The upper posterior synovial pouch was examined with inferolateral approach. Observed were hyperemia and slightly edematous swelling of the synovial membrane, the surface of which looked less shiny and dull yellow.

Case 2 A 42-year-old man with suppurative arthritis of the TM joint (Fig. 202).
The upper posterior synovial pouch was examined with inferolateral approach. On examination, yellowish-white purulent effusion was aspirated. The synovial membrane and villi were significantly swollen, reddened, and also necrotic tissues were observed. After washing out and irrigation with antibiotics, clinical signs subsided.

Case 3 A 44-year-old man with limitation of jaw opening (Fig. 203).
The upper posterior synovial pouch was examined with inferolateral approach. Myeloma of the mandibular ramus was found on the same side. No abnormal findings were observed through arthroscopy.

Case 4 A 60-year-old man with limitation of jaw opening (Fig. 204).
The upper posterior synovial pouch was examined with inferolateral approach. No past injury had been suffered. The synovial pouches were observed to have a marked proliferation of feather-like and slender synovial villi. The articular surfaces of the

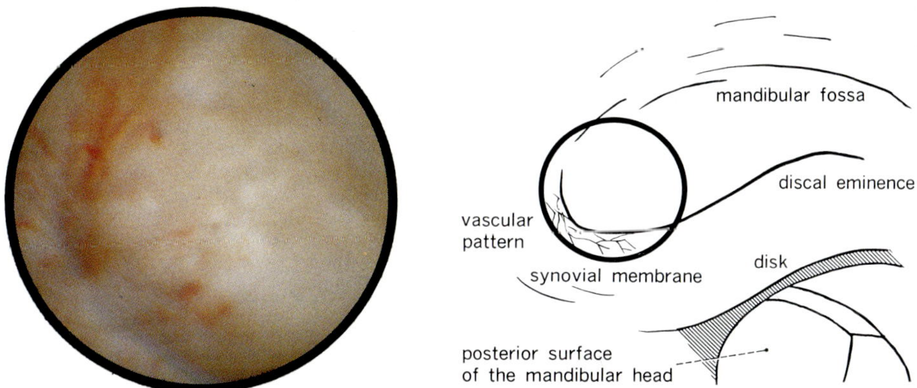

Fig. 201 Subacute traumatic arthritis.

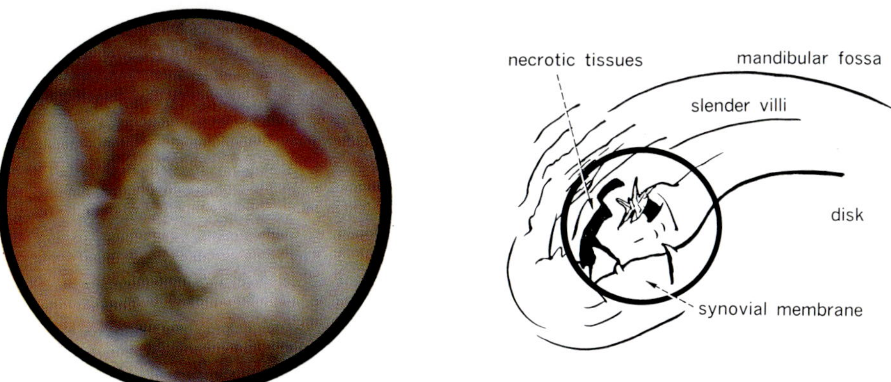

Fig. 202 Suppurative arthritis.

mandibular fossa and the articular disk were also examined, revealing significant fibrous changes. Arthroscopic findings supported a diagnosis of fibrosis of articular capsule of the TM joint.

Case 5 A 68-year-old man with locking of the TM joint (Fig. 205).
The upper posterior synovial pouch and higher intermediate space were examined with an inferolateral approach. Hyperemia and edematous swelling of the upper posterior synovial membrane were observed (a). Normal sliding of the articular disk to the anterior was not seen. Improvement of TM joint locking was achieved through intraarticular ablation of the intermediate space under arthroscopy (b).

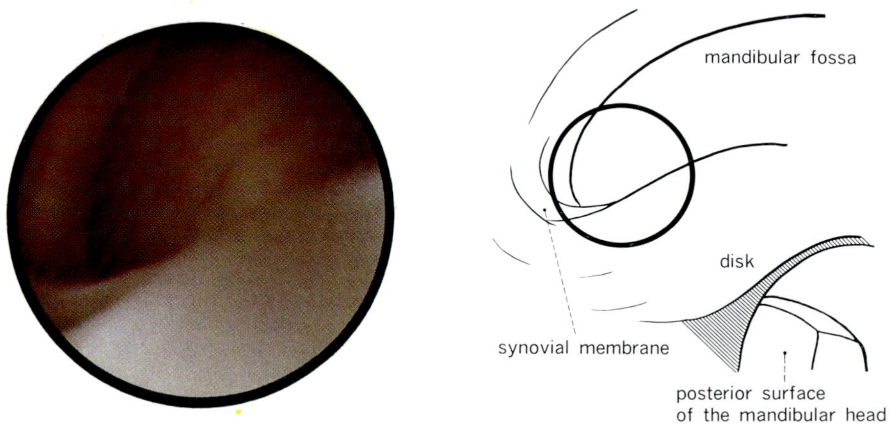

Fig. 203 No abnormal findings observed.

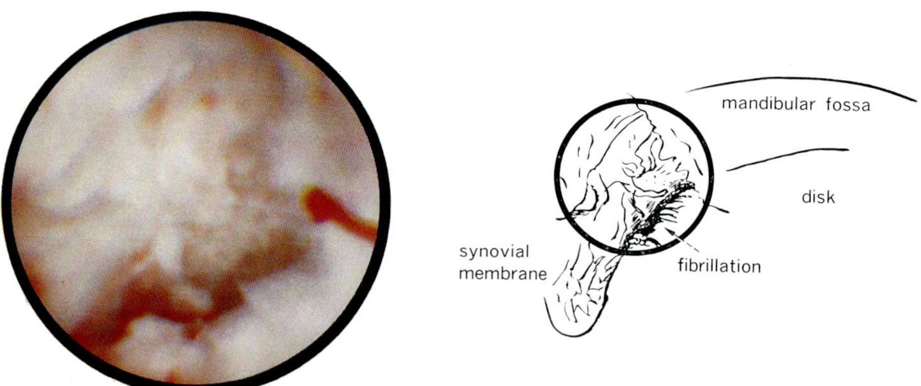

Fig. 204 Fibrosis of articular capsule of the TM joint.

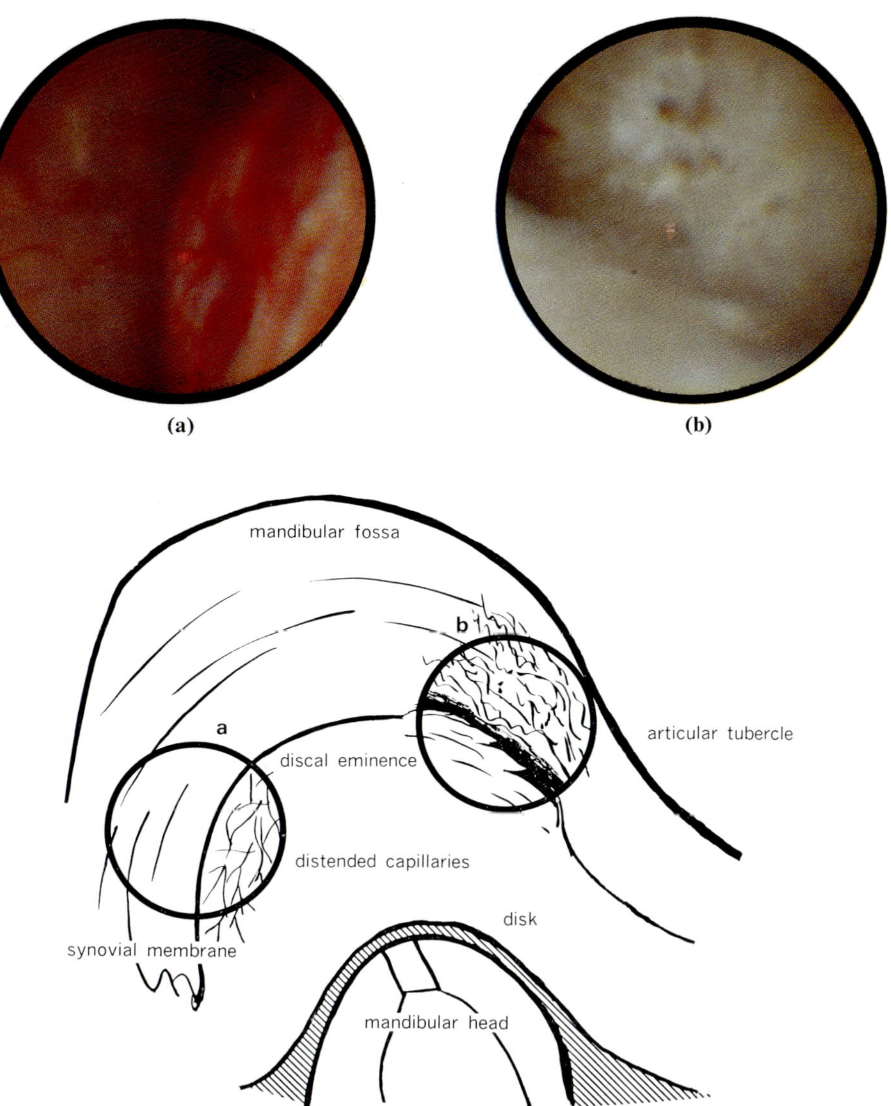

Fig. 205 A case of locking TM joint.

III

NEW TECHNIQUES WITH THE NO.24 ARTHROSCOPY

11

Arthroscopy of the Popliteal Cavity of the Knee Joint

ARTHROSCOPIC ANATOMY

The popliteal cavity is determined anatomically as the cavity lying posterior to the tibial and fibular collateral ligaments. It is divided by the septum into two independent compartments—the lateral and medial compartments. Each compartment is a narrow, curved cavity that can be expanded to allow arthroscopic examination by introducing a sufficient amount of normal saline and bending the knee joint (Figs. 206 and 207).

In 1951, Watanabe observed the popliteal cavity through the anterior approach with a No. 13 arthroscope. Arthroscopic photography was not possible then and findings were sketched by professional artists.

At present, the Watanabe No. 24 (Selfoscope) fore-oblique viewing arthroscope is best

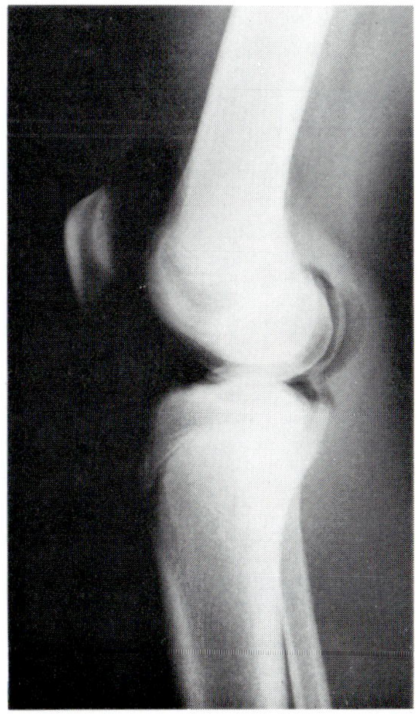

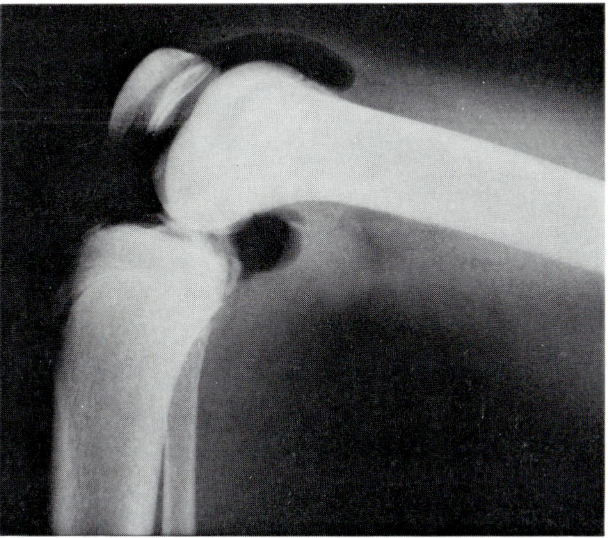

Fig. 207 Right knee joint in 90° flexed position.

Fig. 206 Air arthrogram of the right knee joint, extended position.

for observing the popliteal cavity. The side viewing arthroscope, lately added to the line of the No. 24 arthroscopes, is also very effective when used in conjunction with the fore-oblique viewing arthroscope.

The No. 24 arthroscope was used to observe the knee joints of 152 cases (178 knee joints) from April 1975 to March 1980. Seventy cases (eighty-five knee joints) were observed with the No. 24 arthroscope alone; the rest were observed by a combination of other types of arthroscopes (Table 21).

Anteriorly, it is impossible to examine the entire popliteal cavity by only one approach. Therefore, when necessary, several approaches should be used for a sufficiently through arthroscopic examination of the popliteal cavity. There are eight representative approaches (Fig. 208):

Anteromedial
Anterolateral
Posteromedial
Posterolateral
Medial popliteal
Lateral popliteal
Lateral infrapatellar
Medial infrapatellar

PUNCTURE METHODS

Anteromedial Approach

The knee joint is extended, and the trocar is inserted horizontally (to the medial tibial plateau), anteromedially at about 45° posteriorly (from the frontal plane) at a point just anterior to the tibial collateral ligament, and just superior to the superior surface of the medial meniscus. The trocar is pushed to the outer surface of the capsule, turned toward the sagittal plane, and pushed through the capsule into the knee joint space lying just distal to the medial femoral epicondyle. At insertion into the knee joint cavity, great attention is required to avoid injury to the cartilaginous surface of the medial femoral condyle or the medial meniscus. Insertion is often done under arthroscopic control, guided by a second arthroscope in the anterior approach. A suitable insertion point is determined by punctur-

Table 21 Classification of cases by approach and method

Approach	Combined arthroscopy: No. 24 and others	No. 24 arthroscope alone
Lateral suprapatellar	20	15
Medial suprapatellar	4	2
Lateral infrapatellar	63	35
Medial infrapatellar	34	14
Anterolateral	2	1
Anteromedial	6	1
Posterolateral	8	4
Posteromedial	27	6
Lateral popliteal	1	0
Medial popliteal	2	0
Unknown	11	7
Total number of knee joints	178	85
Total number of cases	152	70

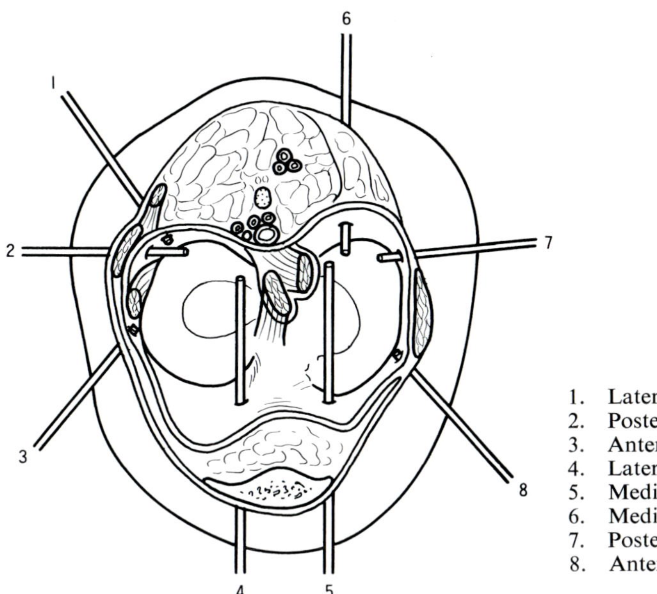

Fig. 208 Eight approaches to the popliteal cavity. (Modified from figure 201, p. 244 in Lang & Wachsmuth: Lanz Praktische Anatomie, I/4, Bein und Statik, 2nd ed., Springer-Verlag, Heidelberg, 1972. Used by permission from the publisher.)

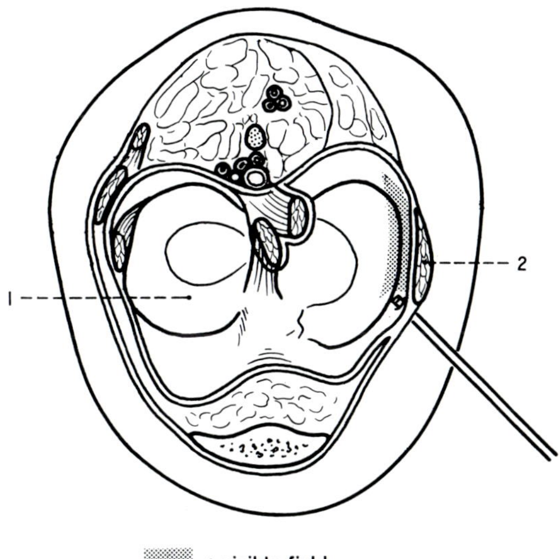

Fig. 209 Visible field in anteromedial approach. (Modified from figure 201, p. 244 in Lang & Wachsmuth: Lanz Praktische Anatomie, I/4, Bein und Statik, 2nd ed., Springer-Verlag, Heidelberg, 1972. Used by permission from the publisher.)

ing the capsule with a syringe needle just superior to the medial meniscus, a point where the No. 24 may easily be operated. The No. 24 trocar is then inserted.

The peripheral rim and the parameniscal area of the medial meniscus, from the medial to the posterior segment, and the capsule are observed (Fig. 209). The place where the medial meniscus joins the capsule is concave and covered by fascicled synovial villi, which sometimes obstruct the visual field.

Arthroscopy is performed with the knee joint valgus, either bent or extended, with the lower extremity rotated either internally or externally. When the knee is extended, the arthroscope can be introduced into the posterior part of the popliteal cavity, but the movement of the arthroscope gradually becomes limited and difficult. When the knee is flexed, the cavity narrows, and the arthroscope should be moved backward gently to avoid damaging the arthroscope.

In cases where the parameniscal area of the medial segment of the medial meniscus is completely torn, the trocar reaches directly to the articular surface of the tibial plateau through the torn portion. Care must be taken to avoid mistaking the articular surface of the tibial plateau for the medial meniscus (Fig. 210).

Anterolateral Approach

The knee joint is flexed to about 30°. The trocar puncture is made just anterior to the fibular collateral ligament and just proximal to the lateral joint line. Taking care to avoid injury to the lateral meniscus, the trocar is inserted horizontally and anterolaterally at about 45°.

The main visualized structures are situated in the section from the middle segment to the posterior segment of the lateral meniscus—the peripheral rim and the parameniscal area of the lateral meniscus and the opening of the popliteal tendon groove (Fig. 211). The place where the lateral meniscus joins the capsule is concave and covered by fascicled synovial villi. The popliteal tendon groove located the popliteus tendon is observed in the section from the middle segment to the posterior segment of the lateral meniscus. Fascicled synovial villi are often seen at the anterior portion of the opening of the popliteal tendon groove, and it is sometimes difficult to observe the shape of the opening. The lateral meniscus and the popliteus tendon require careful observation because a parameniscal tear or scar formation is often observed at these functionally important points. The arthroscope can be pointed parallel along the popliteal tendon groove by withdrawing partially and changing direction distally at about 45°. The arthroscope is guided along the popliteus tendon (Fig. 212), and the inside wall of the popliteal tendon groove is observed (Fig. 213). The arthroscope is gradually pushed further toward the subpopliteal recess. The outlet of the popliteal tendon

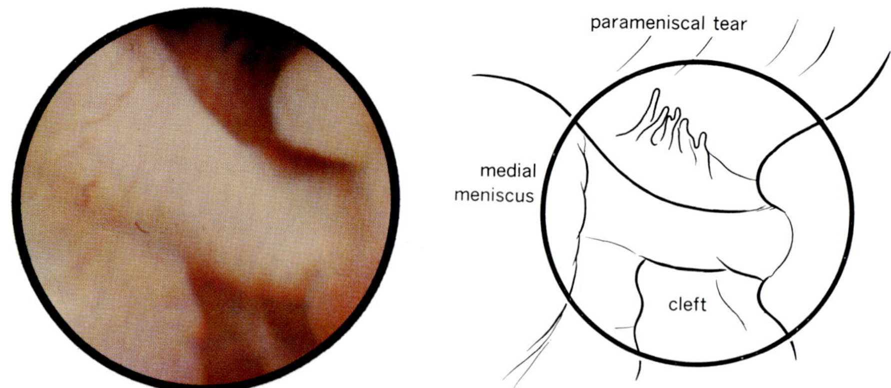

Fig. 210 A 20-year-old woman with parameniscal tear of the right knee joint, examined with the No. 24-C arthroscope.

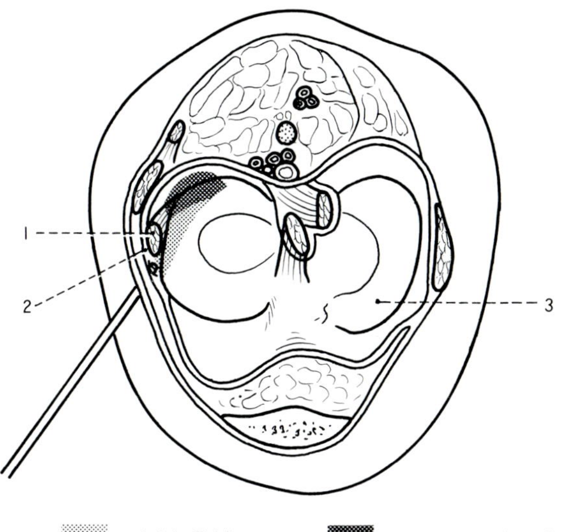

Fig. 211 Visible field in anterolateral approach. (Modified from figure 201, p. 244 in Lang & Wachsmuth: Lanz Praktische Anatomie, I/4, Bein und Statik, 2nd ed., Springer-Verlag, Heidelberg, 1972. Used by permission from the publisher.)

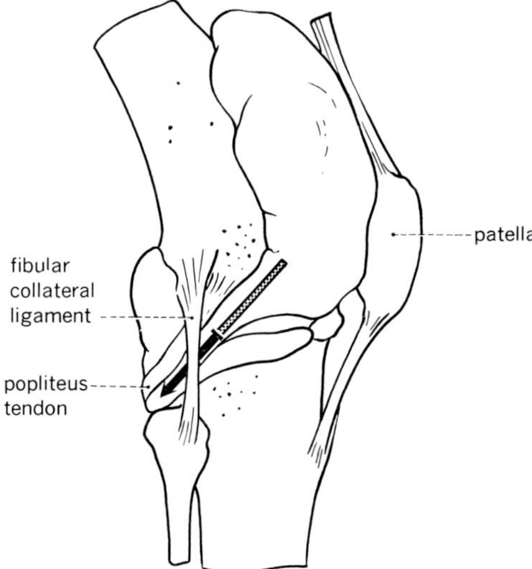

Fig. 212 Anterolateral approach to the subpopliteal recess with the No. 24 arthroscope. (Modified from figure 270 on p. 142 in Spalteholz, W. & Spanner, R.: Handatlas der Anatomie des Menschen, Erster Teil: Bewegungsapparat, 16. Auflage, Scheltema & Holkema, Amsterdam, 1959. Used by permission from the publisher.)

groove, the popliteus tendon, a part of the posterior cartilaginous surface of the lateral tibial condyle, and the inner side of the subpopliteal recess can be observed. One or several loose bodies are sometimes seen in the subpopliteal recess. Slender synovial villi are observed at the anterior part of the outlet of the popliteal tendon groove. The popliteus tendon can be observed on the surface that faces toward the popliteal tendon groove of the lateral meniscus, but the opposite side of the popliteus tendon is concealed by a membranous ligament connecting the popliteus tendon with the lateral part of the lateral meniscus.

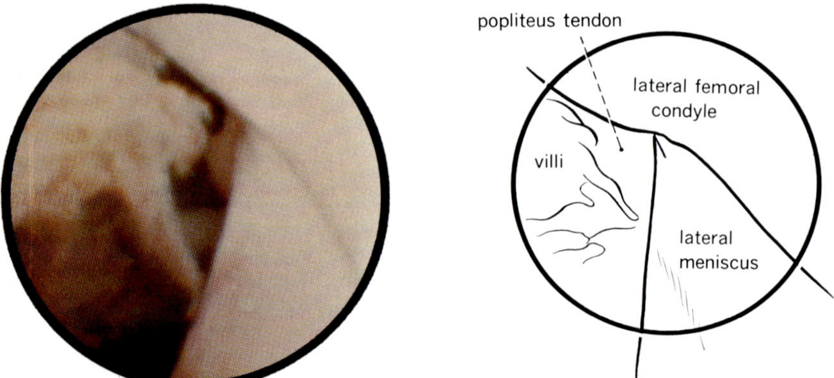

Fig. 213 A 53-year-old woman. Popliteal tendon groove of the right knee joint, examined with the No. 24-B arthroscope.

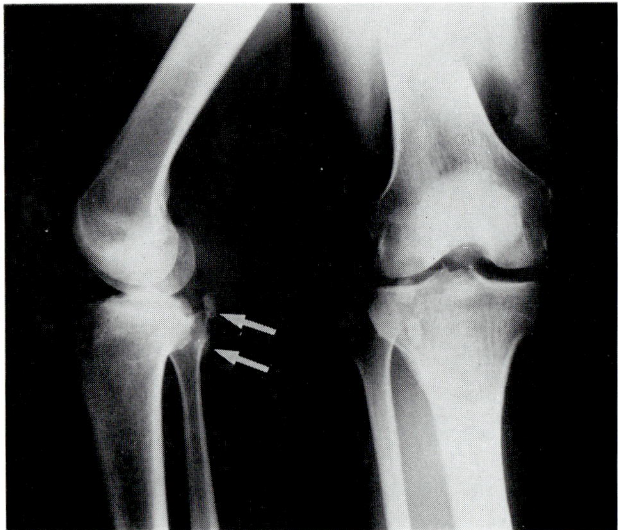

Fig. 214 Loose bodies, indicated by the arrows, in the popliteus bursa.

In rare cases, the popliteal tendon groove is closed by a membranous ligament that blocks access to the subpopliteal recess.

Usually the popliteal vein and artery run behind the popliteus muscle, separate from the subpopliteal recess, and are thus protected. However, it must be remembered that in rare cases the tibial artery can run anterior to the popliteus muscle and is thus vulnerable.

Loose bodies are sometimes found in the subpopliteal recess (Figs. 214 and 215).

Posteromedial Approach

The knee is flexed about 45° in a flexed or cross-legged position. The trocar is inserted posterior to the tibial collateral ligament and anterior to the sartorius tendon, and directed toward the medial popliteal triangular area, which is constructed by the posterior surface of the medial femoral condyle, the posterior segment of the medial meniscus, and the posterior wall of the medial posterior compartment. The medial popliteal triangular area can be easily palpated, especially with the knee joint flexed 90°. Palpation of the medial popliteal

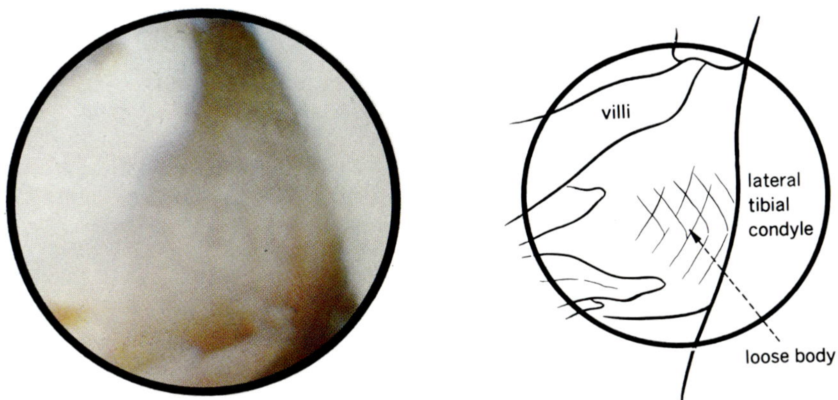

Fig. 215 A 53-year-old woman with a loose body in the right knee joint, examined with the No. 24-B arthroscope.

triangular area becomes difficult with the knee joint at 45° because the sartorius muscle, which slides forward with flexion, lies just across it. After palpation of the medial popliteal triangular area is performed at 90° flexion, the trocar is inserted just anterior to the border of the sartorius muscle, is pushed into the popliteal fascia (the knee remaining flexed 90°), and is inserted into the capsule. This procedure helps the arthroscope move smoothly against the resistance of the soft tissue when arthroscope is performed with the knee extended.

In some cases with exceptional sartorius muscle development, the muscle is situated on the medial popliteal triangular area. Because of its width and thickness, it is unable to slide completely backward, even with the knee fully extended. In such a case, the trocar is inserted into the popliteal cavity just posterior to the posterior border of the sartorius muscle and just anterior to the gracilis muscle at 90° flexion. This avoids injury to the great saphenous vein when inserting through the sartorius muscle.

The standard insertion point for the medial popliteal triangular area is proximal to the joint space, slightly posterior to the posterior part of the medial femoral condyle (Fig. 216). The medial popliteal triangular area is wider and more easily palpable than the lateral area. Insertion can be at any of the preferred points in the medial popliteal triangular area, depending on the desired observation. It is recommended that the trocar be inserted from these points into the medial popliteal cavity only after a syringe needle is inserted to confirm placement relative to the medial popliteal cavity.

This approach allows visualization of many structures in the popliteal cavity. They are: the peripheral rim, parameniscal area of the posterior segment, and posterior portion of the middle segment of the medial meniscus; the posterior horn; the posterior and lower cartilaginous surface of the medial femoral condyle; the posterior curviform wall of the medial posterior compartment; the septum; and part of the posterior cruciate ligament (Fig. 217).

This approach also allows detailed observation of the peripheral rim, the parameniscal area of the posterior segment, and the posterior portion of the middle segment of the medial meniscus, which cannot be seen through anterior approaches. The region where the medial meniscus joins the capsular wall is concave and covered by fascicled synovial villi, which sometimes obstruct the visual field. In some cases, the concave area is a deep trough, i.e., the parameniscal area joins the steep wall of the posterior region of the medial femoral

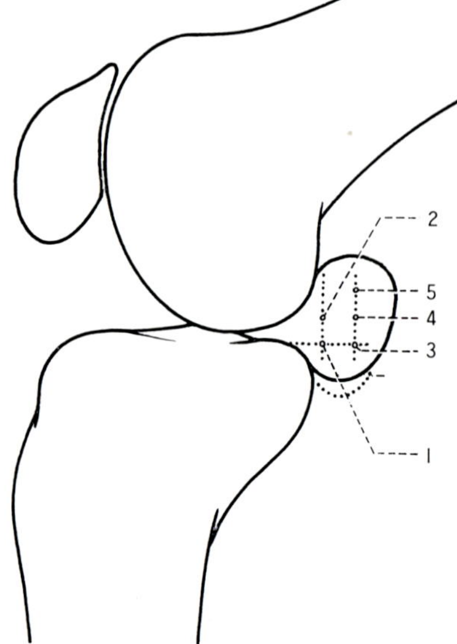

Fig. 216 Puncture points for the medial popliteal triangle. (1) Standard puncture point. (2) Standard puncture point. (3) Puncture point for the posterior cruciate ligament. (4) Puncture point for the peripheral rim and the parameniscal area of the posterior segment of the medial meniscus. (5) Puncture point for the operative apparatus or the trocar.

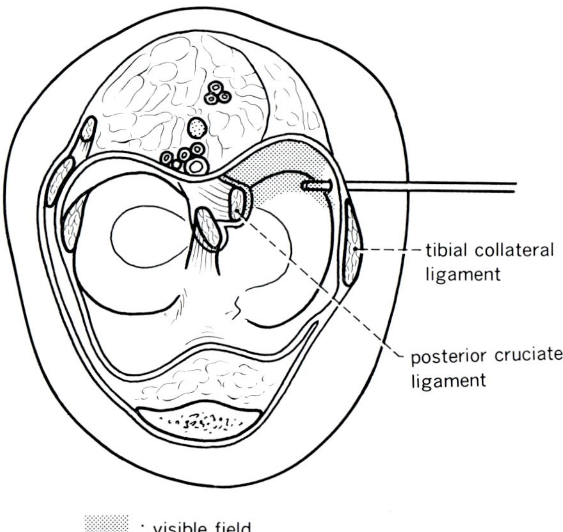

Fig. 217 Visible field in posteromedial approach. (Modified from figure 201, p. 244 in Lang & Wachsmuth: Lanz Praktische Anatomie, I/4, Bein und Statik, 2nd ed., Springer-Verlag, Heidelberg, 1972. Used by permission from the publisher.)

condyle (Fig. 218a). The synovial membrane of the steep wall continues to the bottom of the trough and then turns proximally, constructing the posterior wall of the medial posterior compartment. The synovial villi are fasciculated on the bottom of the trough. The posterior medial popliteal capsular wall surrounds and runs parallel with the convex surface of the posterior medial femoral condyle, constructing a concave form extending proximally, medially, and laterally, and attaching to the proximal border of the posterior medial femoral condyle. Loose bodies are sometimes observed in this deep trough. These bodies are im-

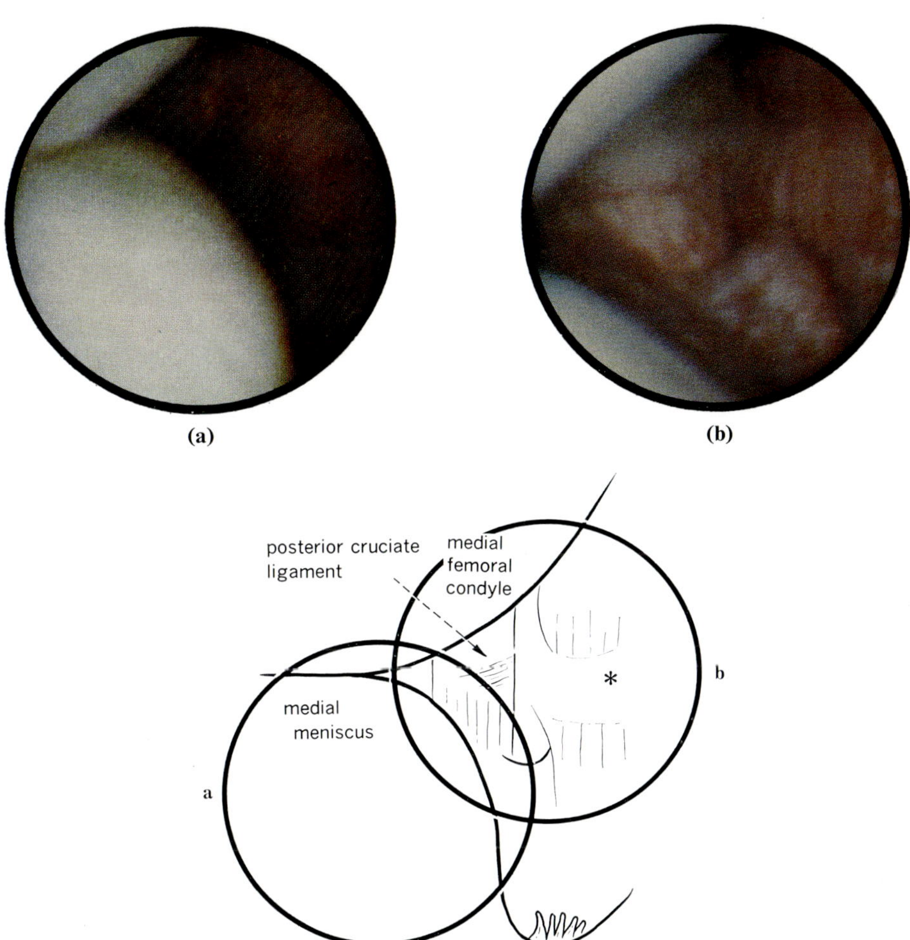

Fig. 218 A 37-year-old man. Right knee joint, examined with the No. 24-B arthroscope. (*) Thin portion of the septum.

mobile regardless of knee joint movement. The slender fore-oblique viewing arthroscope usually cannot observe these bodies through the anterior approaches.

Flexion of the knee helps bring the proximal part of the posterior cartilaginous surface of the medial femoral condyle, and the proximal part of the posterior wall of the medial posterior compartment, into the relatively wide visualized field. The arthroscope is pushed deeply into the medial popliteal cavity, and guided along the medial meniscus to the posterior horn, where the tip is turned to contact the cartilaginous surface of the posterior medial femoral condyle. Then the posterior cruciate ligament, which runs almost vertically, is observed (Fig. 218b). The capsular wall extends posteriorly from the medial meniscus, forming a hemisphere, and then turns anteriorly toward the septum, continuing to the posterior cruciate ligament. The posterior cruciate ligament is covered by synovial membrane. The visualized part of the posterior cruciate ligament includes the medial and posteromedial aspect of the posterior cruciate ligament. The posterior cruciate ligament can be observed through the synovial membrane, as can the anterior cruciate ligament. The vascular nets are usually observed on the surface of the posterior cruciate ligament, but cannot be seen in cases where the synovial membrane is thickened or covered with fascicled synovial villi. The posterior cruciate ligament is moved into the intercondylar notch by extending the knee. Visualization of the posterior cruciate ligament is blocked by the medial femoral condyle, with only the part adjacent to the tibial insertion sometimes visible with the knee extended. Flexion of the knee helps bring the proximal part of the posterior cruciate ligament into view, and 90° flexion obtains the widest visualized field of the posterior cruciate ligament. Increasing flexion more than 90° gradually decreases the visualized field of the posterior cruciate ligament.

With the knee flexed, the posterior portions of the lateral and medial popliteal compartments are enlarged. Also, the septum stretches posteriorly and narrows, with the synovial membranes of the lateral and medial compartments almost touching at the narrowest point of the septum, posterior to the posterior cruciate ligament. The medial popliteal cavity never connects with the lateral popliteal cavity through the septum. In a traumatic avulsion fracture of the posterior cruciate ligament, the lateral and the medial popliteal cavities connect through the broken septum, which normally is adjacent to the posterior cruciate ligament.

Posterolateral Approach

The knee is flexed about 30°. The trocar is inserted horizontally just proximal to the lateral joint space, posterior to the fibular collateral ligament, and anterior to the biceps tendon. The trocar is inserted into the lateral popliteal triangular area, which is constructed by the posterior surface of the lateral femoral condyle, the posterior region of the lateral meniscus, and the posterior wall of the lateral posterior compartment. As the lateral popliteal triangular space is difficult to palpate in obese patients, a syringe needle is inserted to confirm the location of the lateral posterior compartment—normal saline introduced into the knee joint cavity will jet out. After this procedure, the trocar can be inserted into the lateral popliteal triangular space.

After the trocar is inserted into the popliteal fascia, the knee is flexed 90° and the trocar is inserted into the capsule. Care must be taken to insert the trocar posterior to the popliteus tendon, to avoid injuring it.

The lateral popliteal triangular area is most easily palpable, with the knee flexed 90°, making insertion of the trocar easiest. The popliteal artery and vein and the tibial and peroneal nerves move farther posteriorly, thus decreasing the risk of damage by the trocar. Therefore, the recommended arthroscopic procedure is to flex the knee 90°, with the foot placed on the operating table next to the buttocks, or with the lower leg hanging over the side of the table. When using this approach for observing knee movement, and the knee is extended less than 30°, the sliding movement of the tendon of the biceps femoris and the popliteal fascia is blocked by the trocar, limiting smooth movement of the arthroscope and sometimes making arthroscopy difficult to perform. Generally, insertion is slightly proximal to the knee joint space, which can be palpated, and slightly posterior to the posterior lateral femoral condyle. An insertion point most suitable for the desired observation may be chosen within the lateral popliteal triangular area along the relatively wide sagittal and horizontal planes. For arthroscopic surgery, a second trocar for the surgical instruments, in addition to that for the arthroscope, can be inserted and established at a suitable point within the lateral popliteal triangular area to facilitate the operation. Visualization through this approach is relatively wide. The visualized structures are the peripheral rim and the parameniscal area of the posterior segment of the lateral meniscus (Fig. 219); the posterior horn of the lateral meniscus; the popliteus tendon; part of the popliteal tendon groove; the posterior and lower cartilaginous surfaces of the lateral femoral condyle; the posterior and

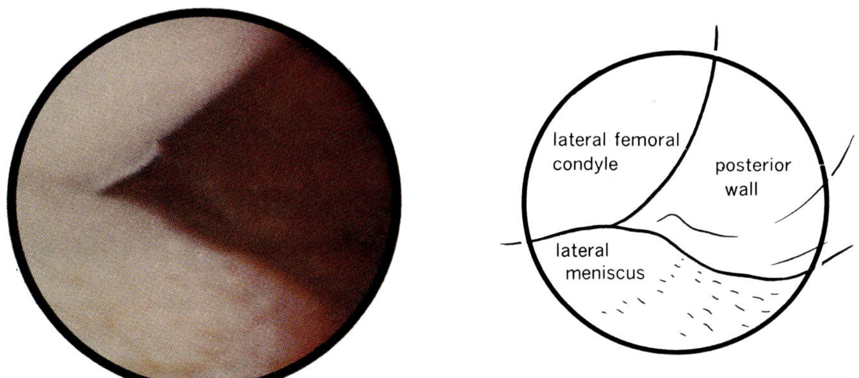

Fig. 219 A 13-year-old boy. Left knee joint, examined with the No. 24-A arthroscope.

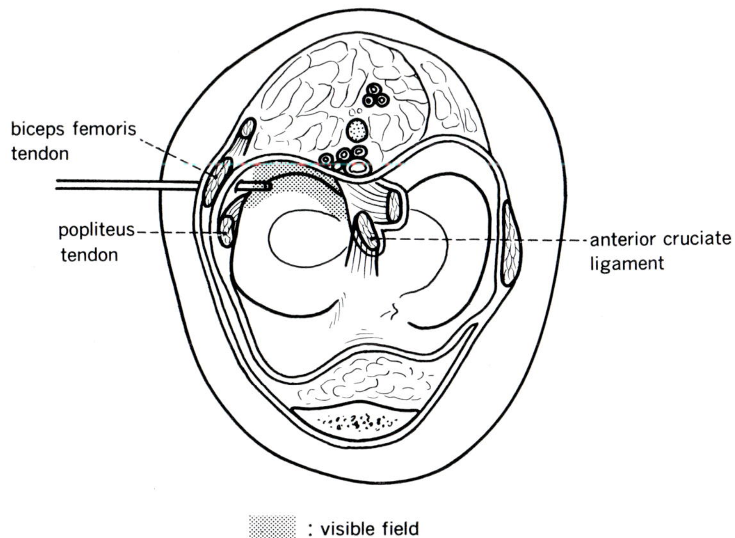

Fig. 220 Visible field in posterolateral approach. (Modified from figure 201, p. 244 in Lang & Wachsmuth: Lanz Praktische Anatomie, I/4, Bein und Statik, 2nd ed. Springer-Verlag, Heidelberg, 1972. Used by permission from the publisher.)

curviform wall parallel to the curve of the lateral femoral condyle of the lateral posterior compartment; and the septum (Fig. 220). Observation of the popliteus tendon and the area near the opening of the popliteal tendon groove is limited through this approach because the arthroscope is inserted so near these structures. At the region where the posterior segment of the lateral meniscus joins the capsule, the connective tissue is coarse and usually it can be depressed easily with a probe. This region is usually concave, and fascicled synovial villi are observed on the surface. In some cases, it is a deep trough and loose bodies are sometimes observed that are immobile regardless of knee joint movement. Even the slender fore-oblique viewing arthroscope cannot observe such loose bodies through the anterior approaches; for such observation, the posterolateral approach described here is indispensable.

The arthroscope is guided along the lateral meniscus to the posterior horn, and sometimes Wrisberg's and Humphry's ligaments can be observed. The capsular wall extends posteriorly from the lateral meniscus, forming hemisphere, and then turns anteriorly toward the septum, continuing to the anterior cruciate ligament. The posterior cruciate ligament is situated just behind the capsular wall in the deepest part of the lateral popliteal compartment, which is lined by the cord from the lateral meniscus or meniscofemoral ligament. It is not connected tightly to the wall—the relief of the posterior cruciate ligament does not appear on the translucent synovial membrane and is not seen through it. However, the deep area of the lateral popliteal compartment should be carefully observed, as it is the nearest possible lateral position to the posterior cruciate ligament. The posterior lateral popliteal capsular wall surrounds and runs parallel with the convex surface of the posterior lateral femoral condyle, constructing a concave form extending proximally, medially, and laterally and attaching to the proximal border of the posterior lateral femoral condyle.

A relatively wide visual field for the posterior lateral popliteal capsular wall can be obtained by moving the arthroscope proximally while increasing flexion of the knee joint. For observation of the posterior articular surface of the lateral femoral condyle, the visualized field can be made relatively wide if arthroscope movement accompanies movement of the knee joint. This reduces resistance by the soft tissue and allows freer movement than if the operator moves only the arthroscope.

Medial Popliteal Approach

A prone or lateral position is recommended for this approach and the knee is lightly flexed. The trocar is inserted horizontally to the medial knee joint line between the semimembranosus and semitendinosus tendons.

The joint space of the medial popliteal cavity is situated almost level with the popliteal sulcus, which is the flexion crease of the popliteal region. It is difficult to determine the medial popliteal joint space accurately through the skin by finger palpation. After estimating the knee joint line by palpating the medial popliteal triangular area, a syringe needle is inserted just proximal to the medial meniscus into the medial popliteal cavity. The proper insertion point for the trocar is confirmed by a jet of saline from the medial popliteal cavity.

Repeated slight extension and flexion of the knee make it possible to distinguish and separate the semimembranosus and semitendinosus tendons with the tip of the operator's finger. Caution is needed to avoid injuring the tendons when the trocar is inserted between them. The trocar then passes just alongside the medial head of the gastrocnemius and passes through the posterior capsule.

The medial popliteal approach provides a wide field of vision. The peripheral rim and the parameniscal area of the medial meniscus; the posterior horn of the medial meniscus; the posterior cruciate ligament; septum; and the posterior and lower cartilaginous surfaces of the medial femoral condyle are observed (Fig. 221). The medial popliteal approach is the most preferred for viewing the posterior cruciate ligament. The medial femoral condyle does not obstruct the visual field for the posterior cruciate ligament, which is situated straight ahead of the arthroscope (Fig. 222). The medial and posteromedial surface of the posterior cruciate ligament is covered by synovial membrane, and a prominent relief rising toward the center of the medial popliteal cavity is formed along the posterior cruciate ligament. This prominent relief constructs a small space in the hemispherical synovial wall, which is situated in the deepest, most posterior part of the medial popliteal cavity. Only the middle portion of the posterior cruciate ligament, about 1.0-cm long, can be observed. Other distal and proximal parts are difficult to observe because the synovial membrane is not fixed tightly to the posterior cruciate ligament and it cannot be seen through the synovial membrane. The proximal part of the midportion of the posterior cruciate ligament is usually

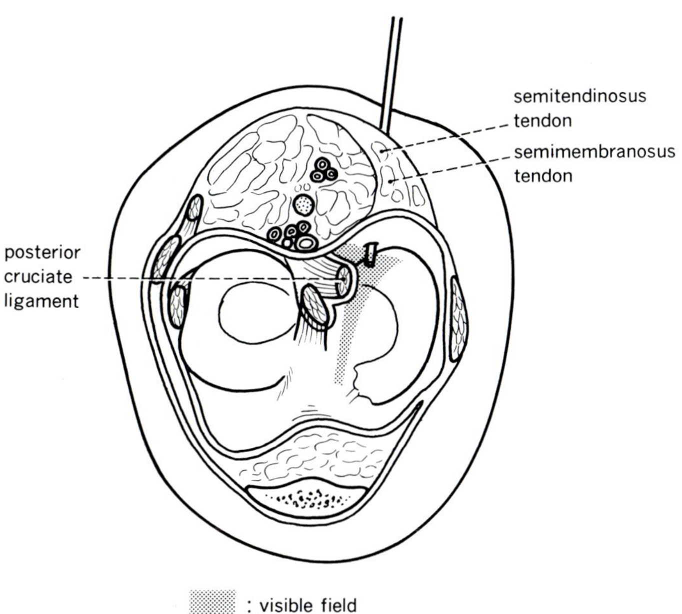

Fig. 221 Visible field in medial popliteal approach. (Modified from figure 201, p. 244 in Lang & Wachsmuth: Lanz Praktische Anatomie, I/4, Bein und Statik, 2nd ed., Springer-Verlag, Heidelberg, 1972. Used by permission from the publisher.)

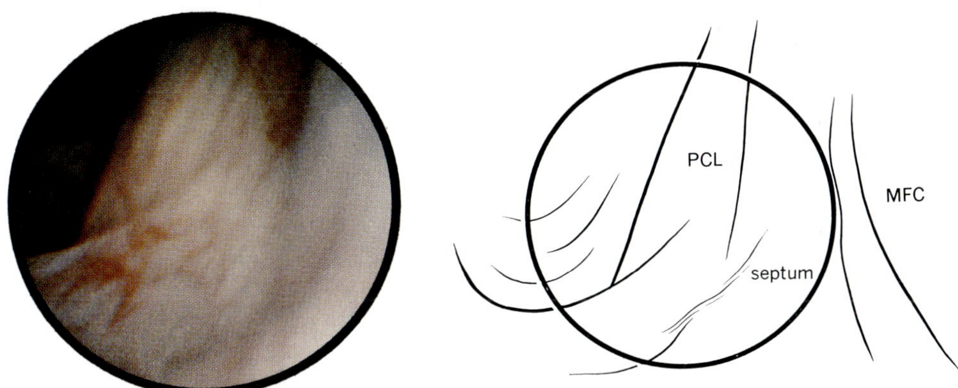

Fig. 222 A 56-year-old woman. Left knee joint, examined with the No. 24-C arthroscope. (MFC) Medial femoral condyle. (PCL) Posterior cruciate ligament.

covered with fat tissue and proliferated synovial villi. The distal part of the midportion can be seen toward the bottom of the popliteal cavity until it is hidden by the thin synovial membrane. The middle portion of the posterior cruciate ligament is fixed tightly to the synovial membrane and its tendon-like relief can be seen through the membrane. The vascular net is seen on the surface of the posterior cruciate ligament. In some cases, thickened synovial membrane, fat tissue, and proliferated synovial villi prevent observation of the posterior cruciate ligament. In the case of a repaired posterior cruciate ligament, the surface of the posterior cruciate ligament is covered by granulation and its tendinous surface cannot be observed. The tip of the arthroscope may be used as a probe to obtain information on the condition of a repaired posterior cruciate ligament, including its adhesion, anatomic position, direction, and tightness. Arthroscopy is performed from the posterior segment to the middle segment of the medial meniscus, but the resistence of the soft tissue reduces the movement of the arthroscope. Also, increasing distortion of the normally spherical visual field of the No. 24 arthroscope occurs near the junction of the posterior and middle segment of the medial meniscus. This distortion of the visual field, caused by bending of the arthroscope's stainless steel tube, is a warning that the arthroscope may soon break.

The arthroscope can be guided forward through the space between the septum continuing from the posterior cruciate ligament and the medial femoral condyle. Though fat tissue and synovial villi exist in this space, the arthroscope can easily advance without resistance to permit observation of part of the fat pad at the medial infrapatellar region.

The posterior articular cartilaginous surface of the medial femoral condyle can be observed in detail, as it is situated straight ahead of the arthroscope. Arthroscopy is performed with passive movement of the knee joint, and is easily done when the popliteal capsule is sufficiently expanded by normal saline. The arthroscope can easily slip out from the popliteal capsule, and care must be taken not to pull it carelessly.

Lateral Popliteal Approach

A prone or lateral position is needed for this approach. The knee is flexed about 30°. The trocar is inserted into the joint just posterior to the biceps femoris tendon at the level of the joint line. If the subcutaneous fat is thin, the common peroneal nerve can be easily palpated along its course through the skin. The common peroneal nerve is not bound so tightly by the connective tissue; flexion of the knee releases the tension on the common peroneal nerve, allowing it to be distinguished and separated from the biceps femoris tendon by the tip of the operator's finger. The trocar is inserted into the joint at a point just adjacent to the posteromedial border of the biceps femoris tendon to avoid injuring the common peroneal nerve. If the common peroneal nerve and the posteromedial border of the biceps femoris tendon cannot be distinctly confirmed by palpation, a small skin incision is made to confirm the nerve and manipulate it medially to avoid its injury. The joint line of the lateral popliteal cavity is situated about 1.0 cm distally from the popliteal sulcus. As the joint line cannot be distinctly palpated through the skin, it is determined by the height of the lateral popliteal triangular area. The insertion point of the trocar is confirmed by inserting a syringe needle, to avoid injuring the lateral meniscus and the articular cartilage. The trocar is inserted just posterior to the biceps femoris tendon until it just reaches the capsule; then the trocar is directed anteromedially, inserted into the popliteal cavity, and pushed along the convex articular surface of the lateral femoral condyle.

The visible field is relatively wide and the visualized structures are the posterior horn of the lateral meniscus; the peripheral rim and the parameniscal area of the posterior segment (Fig. 223); the junction between the posterior segment and middle segment; the posterior part of the opening of the popliteal tendon groove; the popliteus tendon; the septum; and the posterior and lower cartilaginous surface of the lateral femoral condyle (Fig. 224). This approach allows detailed visualization of the area from the posterior part of the opening of the popliteal tendon groove to the parameniscal area of the posterior segment, which is hidden by the popliteus tendon through the anterolateral approach. The posteromedial surface of the popliteus tendon can be observed through the synovial membrane. The posterior and lower articular surfaces can be observed almost straight ahead of the arthroscope. The lateral popliteal approach does not allow arthroscopy to proceed to the space between the lateral femoral condyle and the septum.

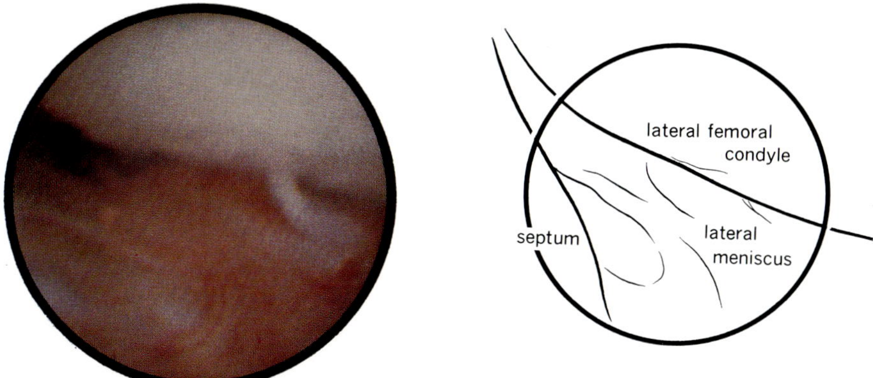

Fig. 223 A 34-year-old woman. Right knee joint, examined with the No. 24-A arthroscope. Meniscorisis was performed at the middle segment of the lateral meniscus nine years previously.

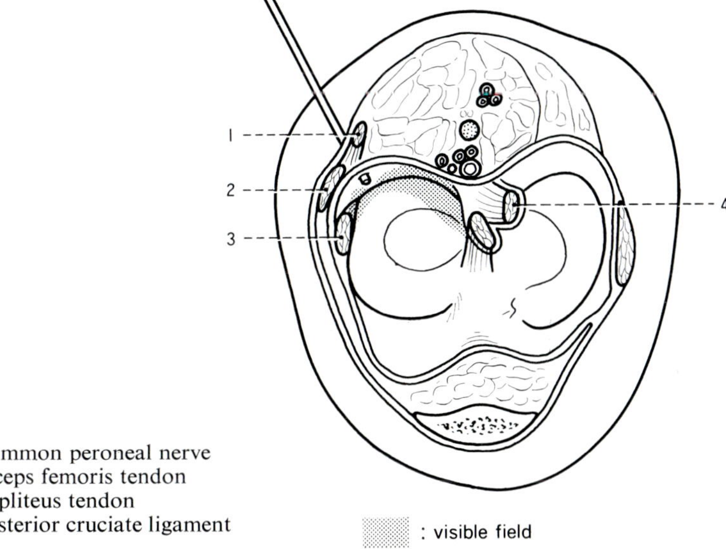

Fig. 224 Visible field in lateral popliteal approach. (Modified from figure 201, p. 244 in Lang & Wachsmuth: Lanz Praktische Anatomie, I/4, Bein und Statik, 2nd ed., Springer-Verlag, Heidelberg, 1972. Used by permission from the publisher.)

Lateral Infrapatellar Approach

The knee is flexed 45° or 90°, with the foot placed on the operating table. The trocar is inserted near the apex of the patella, just lateral to the ligamentum patellae. The trocar is inserted posteriorly, exactly parallel to the articular surface of the tibia. If arthroscopy with the No. 24 is performed just after that with the No. 21 arthroscope, the same insertion route may be used. The arthroscope is inserted into the space constructed by the anterior cruciate ligament, the lateral femoral condyle, and the tibial articular surface. It can easily pass through the space, allowing observation of the fat tissue and the synovial villi, and reaching the medially deepest part of the lateral popliteal cavity, allowing observation of the convex posterior wall beginning from the septum (Fig. 225). If the arthroscope is withdrawn partially, the attachment of the posterior horn of the lateral meniscus to the tibia can be observed laterally in detail, and the peripheral rim and the parameniscal area near the posterior horn can be observed partially.

The use of the No. 24 side viewing arthroscope (Selfoscope) allows observation of almost all regions of the lateral meniscus and the parameniscal area through the lateral infrapatellar approach. The visual angle of the side viewing arthroscope is 90° and the visual field in water is 43°. Because orienting the visualized structures through the side viewing arthroscope is difficult, it is recommended that the fore-oblique viewing arthroscope be used first for orientation. The trocar kept stationary, and the side viewing arthroscope is then introduced into the trocar. This facilitates both arthroscopy and diagnosis. The posterior horn of the lateral meniscus is a good orientation point, and from this point, if the side viewing arthroscope is pushed posteriorly, the parameniscal area of the posterior segment can be observed. As the popliteus tendon is seen in the same visualized field, the parameniscal area and the part of the capsule where the posterior horn and the popliteus tendon join can be seen generally in one visual field and observed longitudinally (Fig. 226). Keeping the popliteus tendon in the visual field, the arthroscope is moved toward it, and the opening of the popliteal tendon groove can be observed. Changing to the fore-oblique viewing arthroscope and keeping the angle of insertion constant, the arthroscope is moved into the meniscotibial joint space. Then, the side viewing arthroscope is again used to observe the popliteus tendon (Fig. 227). At this point, the popliteus tendon runs out of the joint cavity, concealed by the membranous ligament. The appearance of the surface of the popliteus tendon is different from that in the meniscofemoral joint space. The side viewing arthroscope is returned to the meniscofemoral joint space, and the middle segment and its parameniscal area are observed.

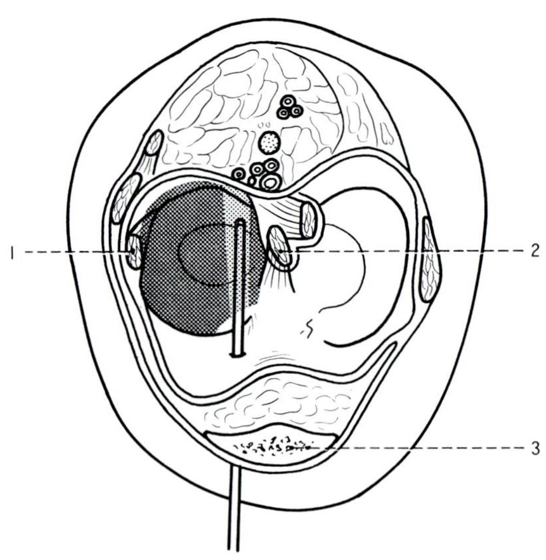

1. Popliteus tendon
2. Anterior cruciate ligament
3. Patella

: fore-oblique viewing arthroscope

: side viewing arthroscope

Fig. 225 Visible field in lateral infrapatellar approach. (Modified from figure 201, p. 244 in Lang & Wachsmuth: Lanz Praktische Anatomie, I/4, Bein und Statik, 2nd ed. Springer-Verlag, Heidelberg, 1972. Used by permission from the publisher.)

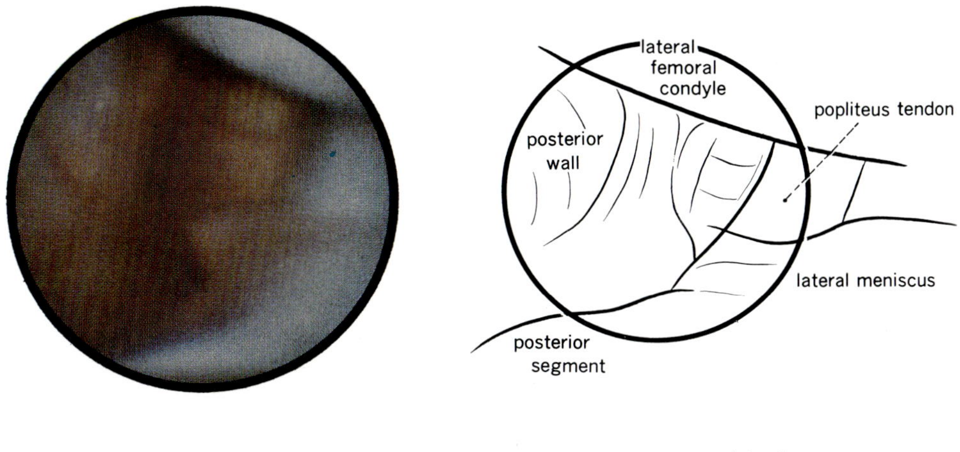

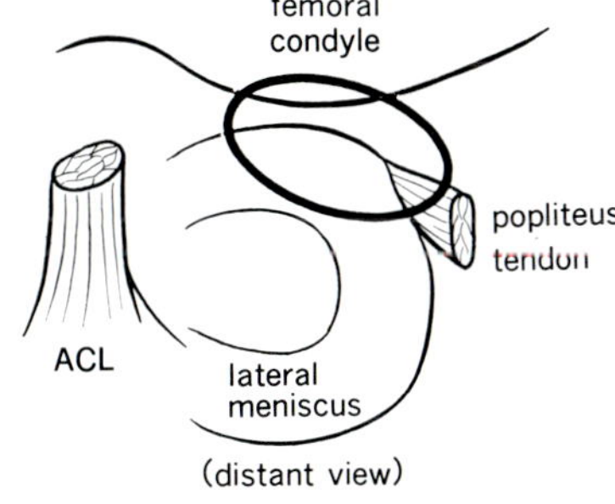

Fig. 226 A 14-year-old girl. Left knee joint, examined with the No. 24-B side viewing arthroscope. (ACL) Anterior cruciate ligament.

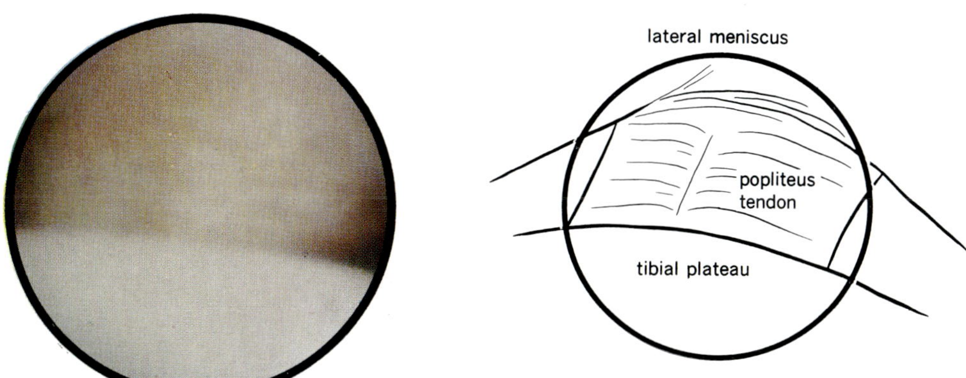

Fig. 227 A 14-year-old girl. Left knee joint, examined with the side viewing No. 24-B arthroscope.

The medial popliteal cavity cannot be observed completely by the lateral infrapatellar approach, even with the side viewing arthroscope, because of lens distortion.

Development of the Watanabe No. 24 side viewing arthroscope (Selfoscope) has enhanced the importance of using the same lateral infrapatellar approach route as with the Watanabe No. 21 arthroscope. It allows general observation of the parameniscal area of the lateral meniscus continuously from the posterior horn to the middle segment.

Medial Infrapatellar Approach

The knee is flexed 45° or 90°, with the foot placed on the operating table. The trocar is inserted within the medial infrapatellar triangular fossa just distal to the apex of the patella and, dividing the width between the femoral epicondyles into thirds, at the junction of the middle and medial thirds. The trocar is set parallel to the medial tibial articular surface, directed exactly posteriorly, and inserted into the capsule. The arthroscope can pass easily through the space constructed by the anterior cruciate ligament, the medial femoral condyle, and the medial tibial articular surface. In this space, fat tissue and synovial villi are observed, as seen in the lateral infrapatellar approach. The arthroscope can easily reach the medial popliteal cavity without resistance from the soft tissue.

The visualized structures are the posterior horn of the medial meniscus, a part of the medial femoral condyle facing the posterior horn, and the hemispherical deep posterolateral capsular wall of the medial popliteal cavity (Fig. 228). Observation of the posterior cruciate ligament is difficult because the distance between the ligament and the objective lens of the arthroscope is too small and the space too confined for the arthroscope to move vertically. With the side viewing arthroscope also, the distance between the posterior cruciate ligament and the objective lens of the arthroscope is too small; detailed observation of the visualized segment of the posterior cruciate ligament is difficult due to lens distortion of the magnified, vertically running posterior cruciate ligament (Fig. 229).

Using the side viewing arthroscope, the entire parameniscal area of the medial meniscus can be observed generally. But the lateral popliteal cavity cannot be observed by the side viewing arthroscope through the medial infrapatellar approach because of the likelihood of bending the arthroscope.

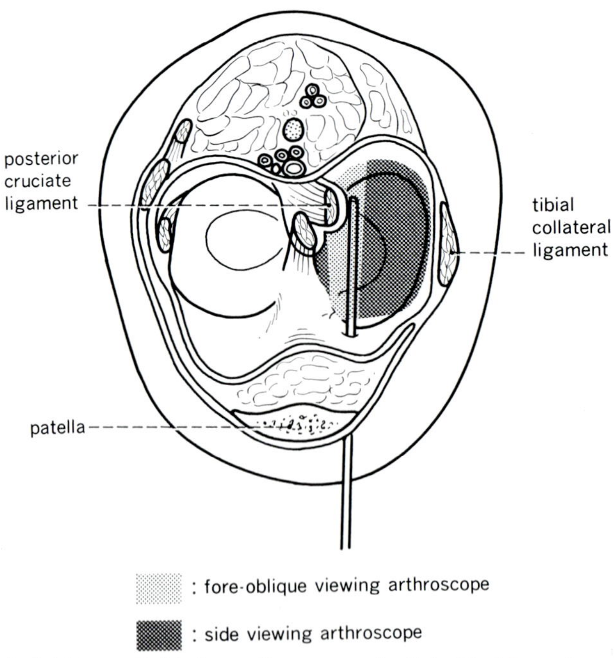

Fig. 228 Visible field in medial infrapatellar approach. (Modified from figure 201, p. 244 in Lang & Wachsmuth: Lanz Praktische Anatomie, I/4, Bein und Statik, 2nd ed., Springer-Verlag, Heidelberg, 1972. Used by permission from the publisher.)

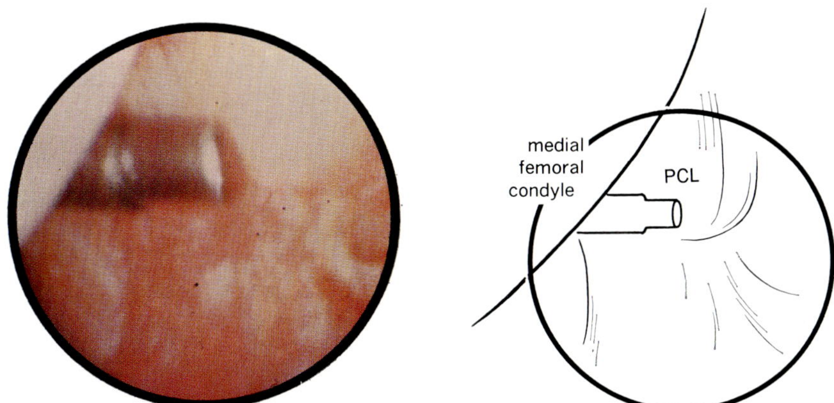

Fig. 229 A 17-year-old boy. Right knee joint, examined with the No. 24-B side viewing arthroscope. The scope is inserted into the medial popliteal cavity through the medial infrapatellar approach, as viewed from the posteromedial approach. (PCL) Posterior cruciate ligament.

12

Tunnel Endoscopy

Tunnel endoscopy is a new endoscopic technique that allows visual examination and surgical treatment of neurovascular bundles, muscles, tendons, and other deep tissues.

Several points concerning tunnel endoscopy were investigated by an experimental study on rabbits. The method was then applied in clinical cases. In most cases, the tunnel endoscopic findings were confirmed by open surgery following the endoscopy. Tunnel endoscopy is now applied to both diagnostic and some surgical procedures.

MATERIALS AND METHODS

Endoscopes used for tunnel endoscopy are the Watanabe No. 24 arthroscope (A, B, C, and D), the No. 31, the No. 21 CLM, the Wolf arthroscope, and the Watanabe biopsy punch with eye guidance. Any cold-light endoscope can be used if its diameter is suitable for the target site. New instruments are being developed.

In most cases, conduction anesthesia is applied because of plans to operate later or to use a pneumatic tourniquet. But, if the target site is not deep or the aim is only observation or a small biopsy, local infiltration anesthesia may be used.

Selection of the approach is critical. It should be based on a knowledge of anatomy to avoid injuries to neurovascular bundles and tendons.

As there is no original body cavity at the target site of tunnel endoscopy, space must be made for observation. At first, the author attempted to dilate the space by injecting air or normal saline (Fig. 230A), but this usually caused emphysema or edema. These problems hamper observation though they can be overcome without difficulty. However, this method has not been abandoned.

Endoscopic Technique

The technique now used by the author is as follows (Fig. 230B). Through a small skin incision, a trocar, larger than the endoscope is inserted. The trocar needle is then withdrawn and an obturator is introduced through the sheath. When the tip of the obturator has reached the target site, retraction of the surrounding tissues is accomplished by manipulating the tip of the sheath. Next, the obturator is pulled out and a small piece of gauze to absorb the blood is inserted by using a slender punch. A pneumatic tourniquet may be used to avoid bleeding.

The endoscope is then inserted. The tip of the endoscope is withdrawn about 2.0 mm

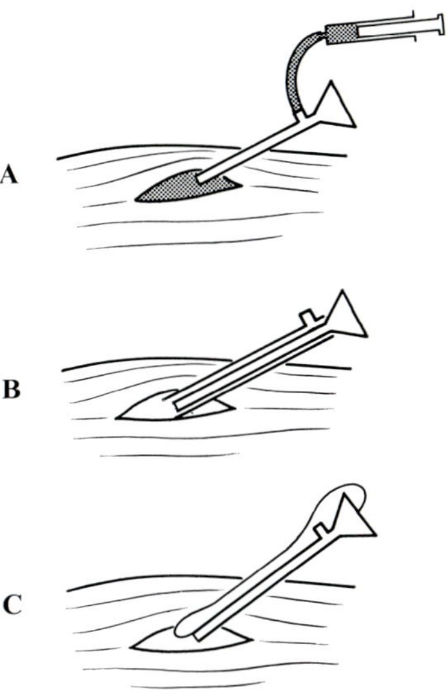

Fig. 230 Various techniques of tunnel endoscopic observation. (A) Tunnel endoscopy with injection of normal saline. (B) Tunnel endoscopy without any medium. (C) Tunnel endoscopy by using a small instrument.

from the tip of the sheath. The space between the tip of the endoscope and the sheath may be used for observation (Fig. 230B). When the target site is deep or difficult to reach, an elevator or some small accessory instrument may be used through the same skin incision with the endoscope to protect it and to provide a better view (Fig. 230C). Operative endoscopes may also be used. A special sheath with an opening device on its tip that functions as a retractor, like the Watanabe biopsy punch with eye guidance, may be used.

CLINICAL CASES

Case 1 A 43-year-old man with rupture of the Achilles tendon accompanied by avulsion fracture of the calcaneus.

On June 10, 1979, the patient fell after running 200 meters. On June 11, 1979, he was admitted to the hospital, and on June 15, tunnel endoscopy and open surgery were performed under epidural anesthesia using a pneumatic tourniquet.

The endoscope was introduced into the Achilles tendon 3 cm proximal to the rupture site (Fig. 231). Tunnel endoscopy revealed a complete rupture of the Achilles tendon. No intact part was observed (Fig. 232). Mingling with the torn tendon fibers was fibrous tissue bundles running transversely. These were connected by white bony tissue at their ends (Fig. 233).

These endoscopic findings were confirmed by open surgery. Suture of the Achilles tendon and Kirschner-wire fixation of the fragment to the calcaneus were performed.

Case 2 A 29-year-old woman with rupture of the left Achilles tendon.

On October 3, 1982, the patient cut her left Achilles tendon while playing badminton. On October 5, 1982, she was admitted to the hospital, and on October 7, 1982, tunnel endoscopic suture of the Achilles tendon was performed under epidural anesthesia using a pneumatic tourniquet (Fig. 234). Figure 235 shows the method used to suture

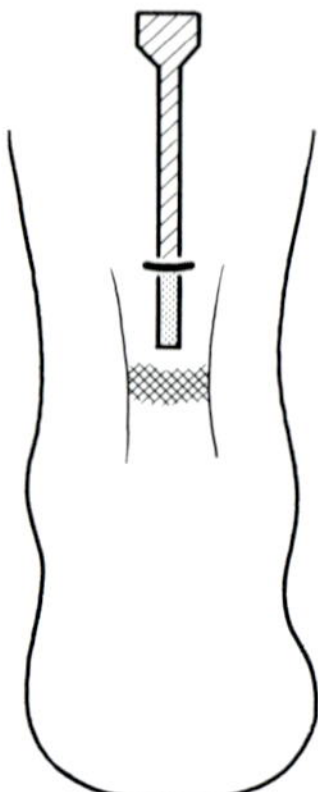

Fig. 231 Case 1. Insertion technique.

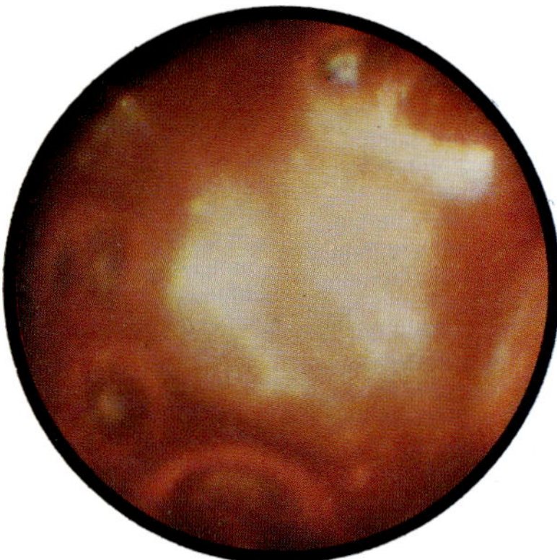

Fig. 232 Case 1. Ruptured tendon tissue.

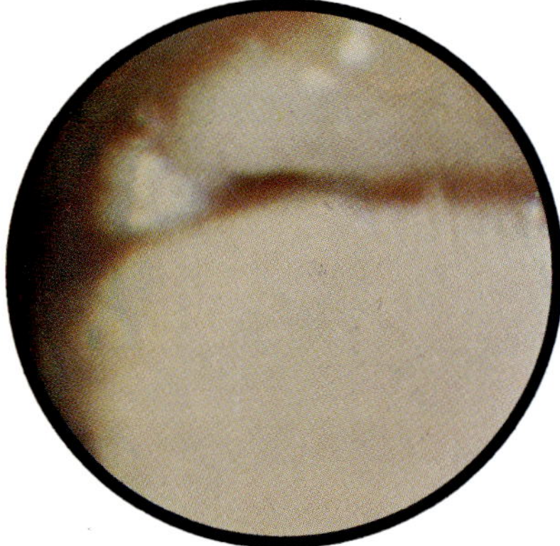

Fig. 233 Case 1. Fiber of the Achilles tendon. Bone fragment can be seen at the end of the fiber.

the tendon. After surgery a below-the-knee plaster cast was applied for about six weeks. Long term follow-up revealed good results.

Case 3 A 28-year-old man with dislocation of the right hip joint with avulsion fracture of the acetablum, and paresis of the right sciatic nerve (Fig. 236).

On August 1, 1979, the patient was hit by a taxi while driving a motorcycle. He was admitted to the hospital on the same day. Hypesthesia of the right leg and anesthesia of the right foot were proved. Muscle power of the gluteal muscle and lower leg muscle were 4 and 0, respectively.

About four hours after the trauma, reduction of the dislocated hip joint was performed under epidural anesthesia. Physical therapy was carried out from the second day. Though sensory disturbance recovered slightly, loss of muscle power remained unchanged.

On September 5, 1979, tunnel endoscopy was performed under epidural anesthesia. A transverse skin incision was made along the gluteal fold and the sciatic nerve was exposed at this level.

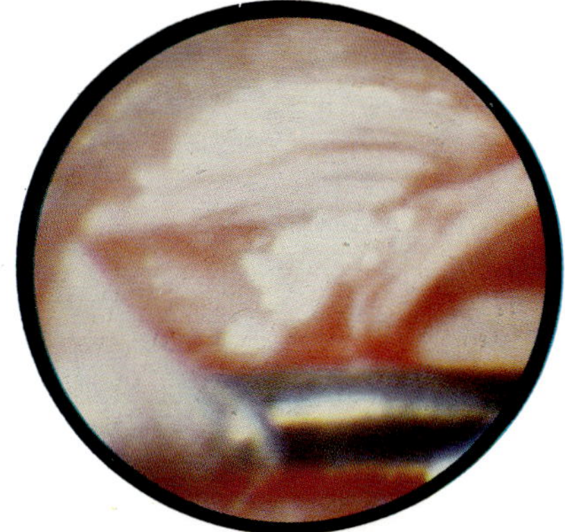

Fig. 234 Case 2. Nylon thread through the ruptured site of the Achilles tendon.

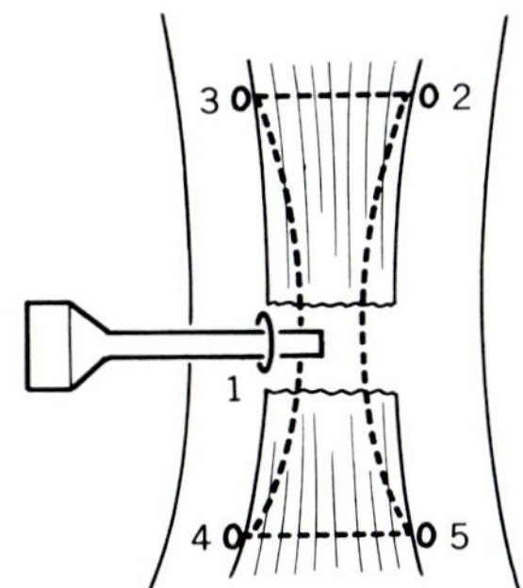

Fig. 235 Case 2. Method for suturing the Achilles tendon. (1) Insertion point of the endoscope. (2–5) Small skinincision to suture. (2) Knotting site of thread. (•••) Course of thread.

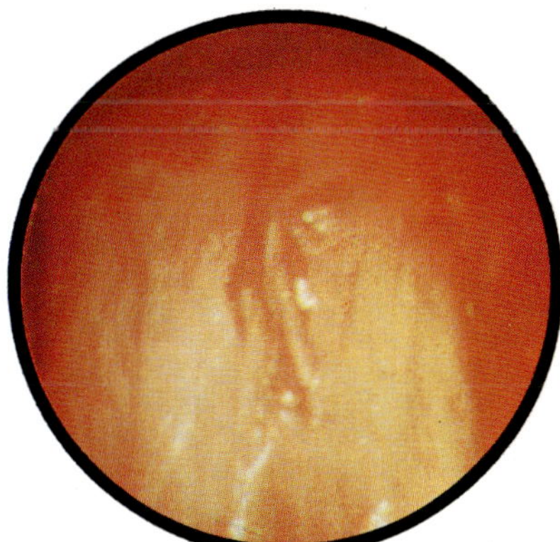

Fig. 236 Case 3. Sciatic nerve.

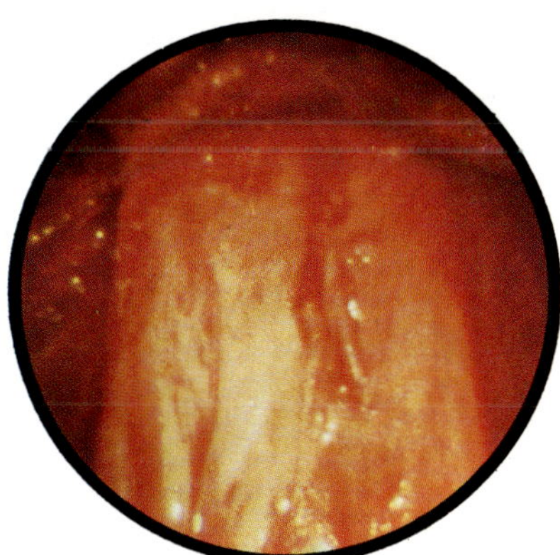

Fig. 237 Case 3. Sciatic nerve, second observation.

Alongside the sciatic nerve, the scope was introduced proximally toward the piriformis, while the gluteal muscle was raised by an elevator. Within the reach of the scope, however, neither rupture of the nerve nor damage by a bone fragment was found. Only color and glossiness of the nerve looked abnormal (Fig. 237). No complications resulting from the tunnel endoscopy were seen.

After two months, the muscle palsy did not show any recovery despite continued physical therapy. A second tunnel endoscopy was carried out by the same approach as before, and neurolysis was performed. The color of the nerve was not good and the glossiness was reduced. At the level of piriformis, the nerve trunk was surrounded by adhesive tissues. Neurolysis was performed and physical therapy was continued (Fig. 238).

The nerve trunk was found to be surrounded by adhesive tissue, and was impossible to see by tunnel endoscopy.

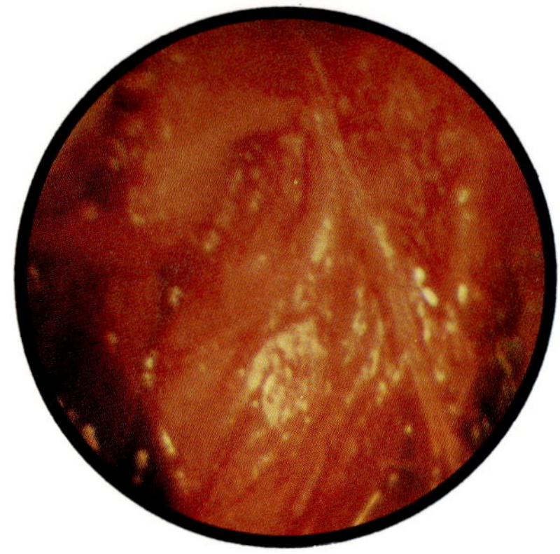

Fig. 238 Case 3. Sciatic nerve beneath the piriformis muscle.

CONCLUSION

Tunnel endoscopy is a new method of endoscopic observation and surgical treatment. Almost all tissues except highly adherent tissues can be observed. With this technique, it is now possible to visually examine and diagnose these tissues. It is useful for making diagnoses, determining surgical techniques, and carrying out biopsies and other small operations.

It is expected tunnel endoscopy will become a more effective diagnostic and therapeutic procedure with the further development of techniques and instruments.

References

Brantigan, O. C.: Clinical Anatomy. McGraw-Hill Book Co., New York, 1963.

Burman, M. S.: Arthroscopy of the direct visualization of joints: An experimental cadaver study. J. Bone and Joint Surg., 13: 669–695, 1931.

Burman, M. S.: Arthroscopy of the knee joint. J. Bone and Joint Surg., 16: 255–268, 1934.

Chen, Y-C., & Yajima, K.: Monoarticular gouty arthritis of DIP joint of left ring finger in a woman. Kanto J. Orthop. Traumat., 6: 12–15, 1975.

Chen, Y-C.: Clinical and cadaver studies on the ankle joint arthroscopy. J. Jap. Orthop. Ass., 50: 631–651, 1976a.

Chen, Y-C.: Arthroscopy of the ankle joint. Rheumatology, 33: 81–88, 1976b.

Chen, Y-C.: Arthroscopy of the ankle joint. Arthroscopy, 1: 16–19, 1976c.

Chen, Y-C.: Arthroscopic study of the cadaver ankle joint. Arthroscopy, 2: 2–7, 1977.

Chen, Y-C.: Arthroscopy of the wrist and finger joints. Arthroscopy, 3: 6–11, 1978.

Chen, Y-C.: Arthroscopy of the wrist and finger joints. Orthop. Clin. North Amer., 10: 723–733, 1979.

Chen, Y-C., Abe, M., Kiyokawa, H., Togawa, Y., & Mizuno, S.: An arthroscopy case of traumatic arthritis of the MP joint of the thumb. Arthroscopy, 7: 25–27, 1982.

Conti, V.: Arthroscopy in rehabilitation. Orthop. Clin. North Amer., 10: 709–711, 1979.

Crenshaw, A. H. (ed.): Campbell's Operative Orthopedics. 6th ed., Vol. 1, C. V. Mosby, St. Louis, 1980.

Fukuda, K., Matsuno, S., Ishii, S., Sasaki, T., Usui, S., Minami, A., Minami, M., & Nakashita, K.: Arthroscopy of the shoulder disorders. Arthroscopy, 7: 13–17, 1982.

Fujimoto, K.: Arthroscopic findings of the experimental arthritis caused by injection of various disinfectant medicaments. J. Jap. Orthop. Ass., 25: 79–80, 1951.

Ikeuchi, H.: Arthroscopic anatomy of the knee joint. Arthroscopy, 1: 71–78, 1977.

Ikeuchi, H.: Normal arthroscopic findings of the knee joint. Arthroscopy, 2: 57–64, 1977.

Ikeuchi, H.: Arthroscopy of the shoulder joint. Arthroscopy, 3: 1–5, 1978a.

Ikeuchi, H.: Arthroscopy of the sprained ankles. Arthroscopy, 3: 12–16, 1978b.

Ito, K.: The arthroscopic procedure and anatomy of the elbow joint. Arthroscopy, 4: 2–9, 1979.

Ito, K.: Arthroscopy of the elbow joint. J. Jap. Orthop. Ass., 54: 1171–1172, 1980a.

Ito, K.: Arthroscopy of the elbow joint: Cadaver study. Arthroscopy, 5: 9–22, 1980b.

Ito, K.: Arthroscopy of the elbow joint: Clinical study. Arthroscopy, 6: 15–24, 1981.

Johnson, L.: Comprehensive Arthroscopic Examination of the Knee. 1st ed., C. V. Mosby, St. Louis, 1977.

Kaneko, K.: Morphological study of the popliteus muscle. J. Nippon Med. Sch., 33: 213–219, 1966.

Kino, K.: Morphological and structural observation of the synovial membranes and their folds relating to the endoscopic findings in the upper cavity of the human temporomandibular joint. J. Stomatol. Soc. Jap., 47: 98–134, 1980.

Kino, K., Ohnishi, M., Shioda, S., & Ichijo, T.: Morphological observation on the inner surface of the temporomandibular joint: Histological investigation relating to the arthroscopic findings in the upper cavity. Jap. J. Oral. Surg., 27: 1379–1389, 1981.

Koike, F.: Arthroscopic study of experimental suppurative arthritis. J. Jap. Orthop. Ass., 18: 656–659, 1943.

Lang, J., & Wachsmuth, W.: Lanz Praktische Anatomie, I/4. Bein und Statik. Springer-Verlag, Heidelberg, 1972.

Last, R. L.: The popliteus muscle and the lateral meniscus. J. Bone and Joint Surg., 32-B: 93–99, 1950.

Maeda, Y.: Arthroscopy of the elbow joint. Arthroscopy, 5: 5–8, 1980.

Miki, M.: Influence of the temperature and pressure of the medium of the arthroscopic findings of the blood vessels of the synovial membrane. J. Jap. Orthop. Ass., 16: 405–439, 1941.
Moore, D. C.: Regional Block. 4th ed., Charles C. Thomas Publisher, Springfield, Ill., 1969.
Murakami, K., & Ito, K.: Arthroscopy of the temporomandibular joint: Arthroscopic anatomy and arthroscopic approaches in the human cadaver. Arthroscopy, 6: 1–13, 1981.
Murakami, K., & Hoshino, K.: Regional anatomical nomenclature and arthroscopic terminology in human temporomandibular joints. Okajimas Folia Anat. Jap., 58: 745–760, 1982.
Murakami, K., & Ito, K.: Arthroscopy of the temporomandibular joint (2nd report). Arthroscopic anatomy and histological studies of human cadavers. Arthroscopy, 7: 1–7, 1982.
Ohnishi, M.: Arthroscopy of the temporomandibular joint. J. Stomatol. Soc. Jap., 42: 207–213, 1975.
Ohnishi, M.: Clinical application of arthroscopy in the temporomandibular joint diseases. Bull. Tokyo Med. Dent. Univ., 27: 141–150, 1980.
Okamura, T.: An arthroscopic study of the traumatic disorders of the knee joint. J. Jap. Orthrop. Ass., 23: 28–29, 1945.
Ota, H.: Anatomical study of the posterior part of the knee. J. Kumamoto Med. Soc., 32: 496–511, 1958.
Sakakibara, J.: Therapeutic value of arthroscopy in the treatment of rheumatoid arthritis. XIIIth International Congress of Rheumatology. International Congress Series, No. 299, p. 41, 1973. Excerpta Medica, Amsterdam, 1973.
Sato, K.: An arthroscopic study of knee joint injury caused by dull force. J. Jap. Orthop. Ass., 24: 184–186, 1950.
Sato, K.: An arthroscopic study of knee joint injury. J. Jap. Orthop. Ass., 28: 467–474, 1955.
Schaeffer, J. P.: Morris' Human Anatomy. 11th ed., McGraw-Hill Book Co., New York, 1953.
Smillie, J. S.: Injuries of the knee joint. 4th ed., E & S Livingstone, Edinburgh, 1970.
Snell, R. S.: Atlas of Clinical Anatomy. Little, Brown and Company, Boston, 1978.
Spalteholz, W.: Handatlas der Anatomie. 17 Aufl., Teil 1, Scheltema & Holkema N. V., Amsterdam, 1959.
Takagi, K.: The arthroscope. J. Jap. Orthop. Ass., 14: 359–384, 1939a.
Takagi, K.: The arthroscope: The second report. J. Jap. Orthop. Ass., 14: 441–466, 1939b.
Takeda, S., & Sakakibara, J.: Development of a highly sensitive color TV system for arthroscopic examination: The second report. Arthroscopy, 6: 81–82, 1981.
Tsutsui, H., Yamamoto, R., Anraku, I., Morishita, M., Kawauchi, K., Fukushima, T., Ara, H., Mori, Y., & Kuroki, Y.: Arthroscopic approach to shoulder disorders. Arthroscopy, 7: 9–12, 1982.
Watanabe, M.: Arthroscopy of the ankle joint of the horse. J. Jap. Orthop. Ass., 22: 59–60, 1949.
Watanabe, M.: Articular pumping. J. Jap. Orthop., Ass., 24: 30–32, 1950.
Watanabe, M.: Atlas of Arthroscopy. 1st ed., 1975. (private edition).
Watanabe, M., Takeda, S., & Ikeuchi, H.: Atlas of Arthroscopy. 2nd ed., Igaku-Shoin Ltd., Tokyo, 1969.
Watanabe, M., & Nagatsuka, H.: Joint perfusion. J. Jap. Orthop. Ass. 43: 496–497, 1969.
Watanabe, M.: Arthroscopy of small joints. J. Jap. Orthop. Ass., 45: 908, 1971.
Watanabe, M., Takeda, S., Ikeuchi, H., & Sakakibara, J.: Development of the Selfoc-arthroscope. J. Jap. Orthop. Ass., 46: 154, 1972.
Watanabe, M.: Arthroscope, present and future. Surgical Therapy, 26: 73–77, 1972.
Watanabe, M.: Recent advances in arthroscopy. Rhumatologie, H. S., 33: 29-33, 1976.
Watanabe, M., & Hirohata, K. (eds.): Surgery of the Knee Joint. 1st ed., Igaku-Shoin Ltd., Tokyo, 1977.
Watanabe, M., & Takeda, S.: Development of a highly sensitive color TV system for arthroscopic examination: Preliminary report. Arthroscope, 3: 71–72, 1978.,
Watanabe, M., Takeda, S., & Ikeuchi, H.: Atlas of Arthroscopy. 3rd ed., Igaku-Shoin Ltd., Tokyo, 1978.
Watanabe, M.: Arthroscopy: The present state. Orthop. Clin. North Amer., 10: 505–522, 1979.
Whipple, T.: Arthroscopic examination of the knee. J. Bone and Joint Surg., 60-A: 444–453, 1978.
Yajima, K., Maeda, Y., & Nagai, H.: Arthroscopic removal of a loose body in the shoulder joint. Arthroscopy, 7: 19–24, 1982.

Index